PREVENTION'S BEST™
America's #1 Choice for Healthy Living

FAT FIGHTERS

Secrets to Successful Weight Loss

By the Editors of *Prevention* Health Books

RODALE

The information in this book is excerpted from *Fight Fat* (Rodale Inc., 1998).

"What Are Your Appetite Triggers?" on page 44 is excerpted from "The Development and Validation of an Eating Self-Efficacy Scale" by Shirley M. Glynn and Audrey J. Ruderman, which originally appeared in the journal *Cognitive Therapy and Research*, volume 10, number 4. Copyright © 1986. Reprinted by permission of Plenum Publishing Corporation.

Prevention's Best is a trademark and *Prevention Health Books* is a registered trademark of Rodale Inc.

FAT FIGHTERS

Cover Designer: Anne Twomey
Book Designer: Keith Biery

ISBN 0-312-97706-9   paperback

Printed in the United States of America

Rodale/St. Martin's Paperbacks edition published January 2001

St. Martin's Paperbacks are published by St. Martin's Press, 175 Fifth Avenue, New York, NY 10010.

10 9 8 7 6 5 4

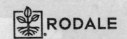

RODALE

WE INSPIRE AND ENABLE PEOPLE TO IMPROVE
THEIR LIVES AND THE WORLD AROUND THEM

Notice

This book is intended as a reference volume only, not as a medical manual. The information given here is designed to help you make informed decisions about your health. It is not intended as a substitute for any treatment that may have been prescribed by your doctor. If you suspect that you have a medical problem, we urge you to seek competent medical help.

Jean L. Fourcroy, M.D., Ph.D.
Past president of the American Medical Women's Association (AMWA) and past president of the National Council of Women's Health in New York City

Clarita E. Herrera, M.D.
Clinical instructor in primary care at the New York Medical College in Valhalla and associate attending physician at Lenox Hill Hospital in New York City

Debra Ruth Judelson, M.D.
Senior partner with the Cardiovascular Medical Group of Southern California in Beverly Hills, fellow of the American College of Cardiology, and past president of the American Medical Women's Association (AMWA)

JoAnn E. Manson, M.D.
Associate professor of medicine at Harvard Medical School and codirector of women's health at Brigham and Women's Hospital in Boston

Mary Lake Polan, M.D., Ph.D.
Professor and chair of the department of gynecology and obstetrics at Stanford University School of Medicine

Elizabeth Lee Vliet, M.D.
Founder and medical director of HER Place: Health Enhancement and Renewal for Women and clinical associate professor in the department of family and community medicine at the University of Arizona College of Medicine in Tucson

Lila Amdurska Wallis, M.D., M.A.C.P.
Clinical professor of medicine at Cornell University Medical College in New York City, past president of the American Medical Women's Association (AMWA), founding president of the National Council on Women's Health, director of continuing medical education programs for physicians, and Master and Laureate of the American College of Physicians

Carla Wolper, R.D.
Nutritionist and clinical coordinator at the Obesity Research Center at St. Luke's–Roosevelt Hospital Center in New York City

Contents

Introduction

Do you know how the dictionary defines fat? It calls it "a white or yellowish tissue that forms soft pads between various organs of the body, serves to smooth and round out bodily contours, and furnishes a reserve supply of energy."

That sounds innocent enough—even desirable. Yet, for most of us, fat is the number one health concern. Some of us worry about body fat because we want to lose weight and look and feel better. Others know that consuming too much dietary fat contributes to heart disease, diabetes, certain types of cancer, and other health problems. Regardless of the motivation, we all want practical fat-fighting strategies that work without taking all the taste out of eating or the fun out of life.

Sound like impossible dreams? They aren't. You can lose excess weight without going on a starvation diet or engaging in a high-stress exercise program that takes over every waking hour. And you can regularly eat generous amounts of great-tasting food without putting on the pounds, if it's the right kind of food. In fact, as you'll learn in this book, you can seamlessly add fat-fighting habits to your daily routine so that after a while you never even have to think about them.

Within these pages, you'll find advice from physicians, nutritionists, and other health experts nationwide that will help you lose weight permanently. You'll discover eating plans tailored to dozens of different lifestyles, including *yours*. You'll see workable ideas for exercising on a jam-packed schedule, options for holding the line on hereditary fat, ways to sidestep common weight-loss pitfalls, and much more. Most of all, you'll learn to make fighting fat your long-term lifestyle, not a short-term diet program that regularly slips into and out of your life. This book offers exciting, effective ways to conquer an age-old problem. Let the fat war begin!

PART ONE

Living the
Fat-Fighter's Life

Goodbye, Diet!

Too many of us wear diet blinders. Screening out much of the taste, smell, and enjoyment of food, the blinders leave us focused on how much body fat particular foods will create. So we look at cake and see fat hips. We look at fried chicken and see a bulging belly. We look at cheesecake and see thunder thighs.

Yet if we want to become successful fat fighters, we must discard these blinders. Although we think diets will make us thinner, all they really do in the long run is make us fatter. There are a number of reasons diets fail, according to researchers.

1. Diets make your fat cells fatter. You have about 30 billion fat cells. These cells can grow in size and number, up to 100 billion or so. Diets actually speed this fattening process. "Trying to starve a fat cell only improves its ability to retain fat," says Debra Waterhouse, R.D., a San Francisco nutritionist and author of *Outsmarting the Female Fat Cell.* "Diets act essentially as fitness programs for fat cells: They boost the ability of fat cells to store fat, to take in new fat, and, in some cases, to increase their numbers."

Why? Evolution. Fat cells evolved to keep us alive during times of famine, and they react to a low-calorie diet as just that—famine. Fat cells respond to famine, or calorie restriction, by holding on to the fat they already have and by becoming more aggressive at taking in new fat once the diet is over.

2. Diets mess with your enzymes. Your cells manufacture enzymes, tiny protein molecules that, depending on the type, encourage your body to either burn fat or store fat. Dieting can double the number of fat-storing enzymes and halve the number of fat-burning enzymes.

3. Diets put the brakes on your metabolism. When you diet, you risk starving your body of vital nutrients because nutrient intake is tied to calorie intake. Very low calorie diets can trigger a complex chain of reactions that eventually tells your metabolism to stop burning so many calories. You may initially lose weight after cutting calories, but eventually the pounds become harder to drop. Then, when you start eating normally, it takes your metabolic rate a while to get back up to speed—and you gain weight.

4. Diets make you rebellious. The more you focus on what foods you are allowed to eat and what foods you are not allowed to eat, the more deprived you feel, says Susan Olson, Ph.D., a clinical psychologist and weight-management consultant in Seattle and coauthor of *Keeping It Off: Winning at Weight Loss*. Then you rebel. Instead of eating just a small amount of the "bad" food, you binge, eating well beyond fullness. "If you say you are going on a diet tomorrow, you probably are going to stuff yourself tonight," says Dr. Olson. Such binge eating can actually make you wolf down more food than you normally would without the diet.

Binge eating also makes you store more fat than you

Escape the Starver–Stuffer Syndrome

Anita eats lean during the week and splurges on weekend restaurant meals. That seems sensible, but not only is Anita not losing, her weight is gradually creeping up. Why?

Anita is a classic dieter, severely restricting calories and fat during the week and going hog-wild on weekends. Since Anita undereats all week long, she craves calories and fat by the weekend, and she indulges in everything from cocktails to fettuccine Alfredo to tiramisu. Consequently, she gets little benefit from being "good" all week. Her total weekly calorie intake still outstrips what she burns off.

The fact that Anita always splurges in restaurants is another problem since she has little control over what she eats there. And, like all classic dieters, she views dining out as a celebration, not just another meal, so she eats foods that she wouldn't have eaten at home.

What Anita needs to do is eat sensibly during the week so she's more in control at restaurants. But she still needs to cut back when eating out. If she includes low-fat—not nonfat—foods in her diet and doesn't restrict her calories so severely during the week, she can minimize weekend cravings and have the willpower to pass on desserts and heavy sauces, or at least eat less of them, according to Franca Alphin, R.D., nutrition director at Duke University Diet and Fitness Center in Durham, North Carolina. This way, the pounds will begin to melt—not as fast as a scoop of vanilla ice cream with pie, but they'll melt.

normally would have, had you spread the same number of calories throughout the day. "If you eat more calories than your body can burn in a few hours, the remainder will be stored as fat," says Waterhouse.

5. Diets don't last. You need to change your eating and exercise habits for a lifetime to lose weight and keep it off. By definition, however, diets mean temporary deprivation. So while you may lose a few pounds, once you return to your normal eating habits, the weight returns. "If it doesn't work in the long term—and that's what matters—it's not effective," says Frances Berg, licensed nutritionist, adjunct professor of family wellness at the University of North Dakota School of Medicine and Health Sciences in Grand Forks, and author of *The Health Risks of Weight Loss*.

Diets do more than hamper your weight-loss efforts. They can hamper your health. Restraining your appetite causes stress and anxiety. You end up so preoccupied with dieting that you lose some of your mental sharpness, needing more time to balance your checkbook, forgetting to get milk when you're at the store, and not hitting the brakes as fast as usual when other cars stop suddenly. Even the most modest calorie restriction can lead to low vitamin levels, causing fatigue. Plus, rapid weight loss can make you moody.

The No-Diet Fat-Fighting Plan

Now, don't get discouraged. Okay, dieting doesn't work. Once you give up dieting, however, you'll be ready to embark on a better, easier, more effective way to fight fat forever. Instead of a transitory, quick-fix diet, this sensible plan gives you the ammunition you need to outsmart the craftiest of your fat cells and turn down your appetite. You'll also learn how to use food, exercise, and even your brain to make your body burn more fat and calories in three ways.

1. At rest. The rate at which your body burns calories to complete general day-to-day activities such as breathing, swallowing, and pumping blood is called your basal metabolic rate (BMR). Your BMR slows as you age. In this book, we'll give you numerous ways to keep your BMR running on high.

2. During movement. Every time you use a muscle, whether you're picking up clothes from the floor or climbing a flight of stairs, you burn calories over and above your BMR. To help you burn even more calories, we'll give you doable exercises that easily fit into your hectic schedule.

3. During digestion. Yes, you burn calories just to digest the food you eat. And some foods make you burn more calories than others. We'll let you in on some of the best-kept secrets about fat-burning foods.

You'll learn tons of strategies designed to help you stick with this fat-fighting plan for a lifetime so you can lose the fat and keep it off. Based on the latest research, the plan focuses on basic fat-fighting principles. You'll find them mentioned throughout this book.

Let food happen. Maybe we should affix bumper stickers to our cars that read, "Food happens," suggests Dr. Olson. Too many of us tend to focus excessively on "good" and "bad" foods, which actually hampers attempts at weight loss, she says. The good-food/bad-food focus makes us crave the "bad" foods even more. That's why the first thing you should learn is that there are no bad foods. Sure, you can cut back on dietary fat, but you don't have to give up your favorite foods. To fight fat, you should actually work your treasured fatty dishes into your meal plan and cut back on other fatty foods, the ones you couldn't care less about.

Eat early and often. Unlike most diets, this plan has you eating more, not less. "Frequent eating works with your metabolism, which speeds up a little each time you eat," says Patricia Giblin Wolman, R.D., Ed.D., professor of human nutrition and chair of the department of human nutrition at Winthrop University in Rock Hill, South Carolina. "Also, if you eat regular meals, starting with breakfast, you're less likely to feel ravenously hungry and overeat at any one meal."

Take the work out of working out. Your body was designed for movement. But if you overexercise, you can get fat. Excessive exercise can deplete your body of chromium, a mineral that helps regulate blood sugar. Your body may respond by increasing the production of insulin, which will make you ravenous. Also, since excessive exercise makes you miserable, you may do it for a while, but as with dieting, you'll eventually quit exercising altogether. And you don't burn extra calories by sitting on your rear. We'll show you how to create your own exercise program, one so comfortable that it eliminates excuses. Your program may be as simple as getting up from your desk for a 10-minute walk three or four times a day.

Lift your weight. Of all the calories burned in your body, 50 to 90 percent are burned by your muscles. Weight training can boost your metabolism by building calorie-hungry muscles. But that doesn't translate to hours in a gym. You can do just as well with a weight-lifting routine that can be done at home with dumbbells. And it doesn't take more than an hour a week.

Don't "should" on yourself. You know only too well how you *should* eat and how you *should* exercise, even how you *should* think. The thing is, you really can't "should" yourself into doing anything for a long period of time.

What really helps is to create your own fat-fighting program based on the advice and suggestions you read in this book. Slowly incorporate doable advice into your life. Don't try to force yourself to switch to habits that you are really unwilling to stick with.

The Rest of Your Life

There you have it. No more forbidden foods. No more deprivation. No more guilt. No more impossible exercise routines. Today you have taken the first step toward what will become a lifetime of thin habits. As you read this book, you'll learn more and more ways to live the fatfighter's life. It's a practical plan that actually works.

The Fat Facts

True or false? When your body burns fat during exercise, the fat melts and comes out your pores as sweat.

True or false? When you eat a slice of rich cake, the calories head straight for your hips (or other fatty zone), where they sidle up to fat and make themselves comfy.

Both statements, of course, are false. But if you had even the smallest doubt about the answers, chances are that there's a whole lot more you need to know about how your body makes and uses fat. And knowing the maneuvers this marauding menace uses to sneak up on you is your first defense in winning the fat wars. So let's get armed.

The Making of a Fat Cell

Where do all those calories go when you eat that scrumptious, rich cake?

Once it's been savored by your tastebuds, the cake slides down your throat and goes into your stomach, where digestive juices work on it. Then it moves into your small intestine. Here's where fat and nutrients are absorbed, part and parcel, through the intestinal wall and shipped off through your bloodstream to various cells in your body.

Once in your bloodstream, the fat that you eat is easily converted into body fat. Since a gram of fat carries more calories than a gram of carbohydrate or protein, your body stores fat about twice as easily as it does carbohydrate and protein.

Unfortunately, your body's ability to store fat is nearly limitless. When space in your fat cells gets a little tight, the cells have the ability to grow in size. Fat cells can also multiply. We're all born with a genetically determined number of these cells, but as we grow, our bodies continue to manufacture them until adulthood, when new fat cell production usually stops. By this time, we've accumulated about 30 billion of them, give or take a few million.

Only two things can trigger more fat cell production in adulthood: One is the purely female prerogative of pregnancy. The other is weight gain. Yes, as nasty as it sounds, gaining weight only makes fat cells feistier. But they do give you a bit of a break: They begin to replicate only when you start pushing the scales at more than 160 percent of your ideal weight. So if your normal weight is 130 pounds, you wouldn't start greeting new fat cells until you reached 208 pounds. Once you make a new fat cell, though, you have it for life.

Fat cells are intended as reservoirs for energy, with each pound of captive fat holding 3,500 calories of energy. When your body can't find enough carbohydrate and protein to burn for energy, a fat cell releases a captive glob of fat into the bloodstream, where an enzyme called lipoprotein lipase is waiting to break it down and direct it toward needy cells.

Who Wears the Fat Genes?

When it comes to producing fat cells, women have it all over men, thanks to a heritage that dates back to prehistoric days. During those times, women's primary job was to keep the population growing through breeding. The men's job was to keep the population growing through feeding.

You could argue that women were a lot better at their calling than men. It was a feast-or-famine existence. Many times, while men were gone for days on end, hunting for food, women were left behind with little sustenance other than their own fat stores to protect them and their unborn children from starvation. Women needed extra fat to sustain themselves through pregnancy and nursing, so the female body, because of the times, was conditioned to store it.

"The male fat cell developed so that it could protect one person, its male owner, from starvation during a famine. The female fat cell evolved so that it could protect two, its female owner and her developing fetus," says Debra Waterhouse, R.D., a San Francisco nutritionist and author of *Outsmarting the Female Fat Cell*. "The better a woman's fat-storing ability, the greater the chances that she, and the entire species, would survive. In fact, if the female fat cell hadn't evolved to be so stubborn, we might not be here today."

Today, however, we don't have to go days or months without food, so we probably don't need quite as much fat. Yet our bodies have not adapted.

Because the lower body is a convenient place to store fat for pregnancy, that's where most women carry their fat—on their thighs, hips, and buttocks. Such fat gives many women a pear shape, with narrow shoulders and wider hips.

Most men and some women, on the other hand, tend

to have most of their fat in their abdomens, making them apple-shaped. As opposed to the fat on the thighs, hips, and buttocks, abdominal fat, also called visceral fat, is a "harder" kind of fat that doesn't feel soft and flabby. "Visceral fat is the type of fat associated with diseases like blood sugar problems, adult diabetes, high blood pressure, high blood cholesterol, and heart disease," says Joanne Curran-Celentano, R.D., Ph.D., associate professor of nutritional sciences at the University of New Hampshire in Durham.

Although apple-shaped people are at higher risk for disease, they do have one thing over the pear-shaped ones: They have an easier time losing weight. Abdominal fat is more metabolically active than the fat on the hips and thighs. "It accumulates faster, but it also breaks down faster than fat on the thighs or butt," says Jill Kanaley, Ph.D., assistant professor of exercise physiology at Syracuse University in New York.

Corralling the Fat Cell

So there you have it. Fat is pretty darn durable. But that doesn't mean that it's undefeatable. This book is filled with savvy ways to get rid of fat forever. And a good place to start is with some strategies aimed directly at your fat cells.

Don't starve. When you diet in an attempt to lose weight, you just strengthen your fat cells' ability to retain fat, according to Waterhouse. Women, in particular, strengthen their fat cells by embarking on an average of 10 diets in their lifetimes. When you restrict your calorie intake through dieting, your fat cells believe that you're at risk of starvation. This prompts them to hold on to fat and to accumulate even more fat once you go off your diet. "Diets teach fat cells to defend themselves," says Waterhouse. "The result is a system of fat protection that can be very difficult to crack, especially if the system becomes stronger each time we diet."

Slow down. To lose weight and keep it off, aim for slow losses, not fast ones. A reasonable rate is ½ to 1 pound a week. Slow losses will prevent your fat cells from mounting a defense.

Go 10 weeks at a time. It takes time to break old patterns and establish new ones. If you've been having three pats of butter on your toast every morning and you switch to using a teaspoon of all-fruit spread, for example, it will take weeks before you're used to the new routine. You should pledge your body to 10 weeks of effort, experts advise. If you're still eating low-fat after 10 weeks, you've probably established the healthy new behavior.

Move. Overeating is not the largest problem in obesity—underexercising is. Exercise helps weight loss in three ways. First, it burns calories over and above the number that we would usually burn in one day. Second, it builds muscle, which burns more calories than fatty tissue does. In fact, people who exercise for an hour a day use up about 8 percent more calories than the average couch potato, even while they rest. Finally, exercise conditions your fat-burning enzymes to break down fat faster.

Take advantage of breastfeeding. Women who are of childbearing age and thinking about having a baby should plan to breastfeed instead of bottle-feed. Their bodies will burn tons of calories just in the act of producing the milk. "Not only does it take calories to make the milk, but when the milk is secreted, lots of calories go with it," says Dr. Curran-Celentano.

Check Out Your Genes to Size Up Your Size

Fat isn't fair. It seems as if some people could eat all the time, sit on their rears all day long, snack while they watch TV at night, and indulge in decadent desserts yet never appear to gain an ounce.

On the other hand, it seems that other people could eat hardly anything and watch each crumb they eat. They could walk whenever possible and never eat a thing when watching TV. Yet for them, gaining weight comes as easily as growing hair.

If you fall into the second category, don't blame yourself. It's not necessarily your fault. Blame it on your genes.

The Gene Trap
Yes, a lot of people who struggle with their weight have their ancestors to thank. But don't feel that this gives you license to wave the white flag and reach for a bag of cookies. Your genes may be working against you, but you can fight fat. It's just that you may have to work harder at it than others, says Barbara Hansen, Ph.D., professor of

physiology and director of the obesity and diabetes research center at the University of Maryland School of Medicine in Baltimore.

Historically, someone who was overweight or obese was thought to eat like a glutton. Then studies conducted during the late 1980s and early 1990s began revealing a much different picture, showing that many overweight people did not necessarily eat more than their thinner counterparts. Instead, they had more complicated, biologically seated factors working against them. Here's the evidence.

- Six days a week for 100 days, researchers fed identical twins 1,000 calories more than usual. Even though everyone overate, some eaters gained more weight than others. Within each set of twins, however, the siblings gained similar amounts.
- In a study that looked at identical twins who were raised apart, researchers found that, regardless of eating and exercise habits, the amount of weight gained by each twin was similar to that gained by her sibling.
- In a laboratory, researchers isolated a gene in mice, called the ob gene, that caused increased appetite and slower metabolism. Later, a similar fat gene was found in humans; right now, however, the evidence suggests that it rarely causes obesity in humans.

Although research is just beginning to unravel how our genes may make us fat, scientists speculate that a few different fat genes may have survived from past generations of people who struggled against starvation during times of food scarcity. Such genes allowed those ancestors to eat and store calories when food was plentiful. Then, when food was scarce, the genes helped the people burn fewer

Do Your Genes Fit?

Scientists have not yet perfected tests that would let you give some blood, have it analyzed, and find out whether or not you have fat genes. But they are at the point where they can look at various factors, such as whether or not your parents are fat, and let you know your chances of having a weight problem. Check the following list to discover your genetic lot.

- If both of your parents are overweight, you have an 80 percent chance of also having weight problems.
- If one parent is overweight, your odds are 40 percent.
- If neither parent is overweight, you have only a 10 percent chance of being overweight.
- If you're African-American, you're twice as likely as a Caucasian to be overweight.
- If you're Native American, from the Pacific Islands, or Hispanic, you're likely to have more trouble fighting fat than someone of European ancestry.
- If you're Asian-American, you have less chance of becoming fat than members of other ethnic groups; but beware, because any excess fat will tend to land on your abdomen.

calories so that they could live off their fat as long as needed, thus helping them to survive, researchers theorize. This gene is thought to be especially prevalent among Native Americans, Pacific Islanders, Hispanics, and African-Americans, who seem to store fat more easily than other ethnic groups.

Natural Appetite Suppressants

Did you inherit fat genes? Just take a look at photos of your ancestors, says Dr. Hansen. If you did inherit fat genes, you'll gain weight more easily than those who didn't. You also probably inherited your appetite, your cravings, and your metabolism. Yet fatness is not inevitable. There are ways to turn down your appetite. Here's how.

Eat chocolate. If you do not have diabetes, an allergy, or any other medical condition that prevents you from eating chocolate, small amounts of dark chocolate can encourage your brain to produce serotonin and other feel-good chemicals that suppress hunger, according to Leah J. Dickstein, M.D., professor and associate chair for academic affairs in the department of psychiatry and behavioral sciences at the University of Louisville School of Medicine in Kentucky. Self-medicating with small amounts of dark chocolate works especially well for women just before menstruation, she says. Also, research indicates that the type and proportions of fat in dark chocolate aren't as bad for your heart as other types of fat. As long as you use it in small amounts, it won't wreck your diet.

Don't drink. Alcohol depletes your brain of serotonin, says Dr. Dickstein. So if you don't drink, don't start. And if you do, cut back.

Work off your hunger. Here's one more reason to exercise: It raises serotonin levels, says Dr. Dickstein.

Eat carbohydrates early. In laboratory animals, levels of brain chemicals that stimulate the appetite for carbohydrates peak early in the morning, says Sarah Leibowitz, Ph.D., behavioral neurobiologist at Rockefeller University in New York City. So a high-carbohydrate breakfast may shut off the "eat carbohydrate" message and leave you sated. Try whole wheat pancakes, oatmeal, or cold cereal in the morning, instead of eggs and bacon, she suggests.

Take sugar in small spoonfuls. After you eat carbohydrates, your digestive system breaks them down into simple sugars that enter your bloodstream. When the sugars appear, your pancreas secretes insulin that shuttles the sugar to hungry cells. If you eat too much sugar at one time, however, your pancreas overproduces insulin, making your blood sugar levels plummet. This reaction can leave you feeling tired and irritable and may bring on a craving, says Elizabeth Somer, R.D., nutritionist and author of *Nutrition for Women* and *Food and Mood.* You don't have to cut out of your diet all the sugary foods you love, she says; just don't eat too much of them all at once.

Feast on fiber. Eating soluble fiber will depress your appetite and your body's postmeal insulin response. Normally, insulin levels rise after a meal, but soluble fiber keeps these levels lower. So stock up on barley, corn, oat products, beans, apples, citrus fruits, and root vegetables.

Trick Your Tastebuds

Your lifetime exposure to certain foods determines the majority of your food preferences. If you enjoy broccoli, for instance, it may be because you ate a lot of it as a child, says Dr. Hansen. Many of your food habits are learned early and are influenced by those around you, she says. But your genes do have some influence on the amount of food you crave and how strongly your preferences dictate what you actually eat, she adds. This explains why twins raised apart naturally gravitate toward the same body shape and weight.

Your preference for different foods, however, is actually one of the easier traits to change, says Deborah J. Bowen, Ph.D., psychologist at the Fred Hutchinson Cancer Research Center in Seattle, who is conducting studies on food preferences. She has found that people who avoid high-sugar and high-fat foods lose their taste for them. Here is what you can do.

Give yourself a few months. Changing your eating habits takes time. To reduce the fat in your diet, you must start gradually and be patient. In fact, studies show that it takes about 3 months to derail any habit—and for most people, fat is a habit.

Slowly reduce your consumption of high-fat foods by fighting one fatty food at a time. If you regularly eat fried chicken three times a week, for instance, try to limit your consumption by indulging only once a week. And when you do partake, try oven-baked chicken. At the same time, increase your consumption of fruits, vegetables, and grains. If you eat only one piece of fruit a day, for instance, add an apple at lunch.

Procrastinate. When you feel compelled to have a fatty food, wait 10 minutes. If you are not really hungry, the craving will pass, says Linda Crawford, eating-behavior specialist at Green Mountain at Fox Run, a health and weight-management community in Ludlow, Vermont.

Create a diversion. When you feel a craving coming on, distract yourself by engaging in an activity that requires concentration and prevents eating. Take a walk, ride your bike, surf the Internet, or play with the kids, says Crawford.

Vacate the premises. Distance yourself from food by leaving the scene of the snack. Once out of sight, goodies are often out of mind, says Crawford.

Savor what you like. Decide what amount of the fattening food is reasonable to eat; then nibble on the favored food slowly, savoring every bite. Scarfing ice cream from a ½-gallon container isn't a good idea. Instead, dish out one conservative scoop, satisfy your craving, and then get on with your life.

Rev Your Metabolism

You may not feel as if you burn a ton of calories every time your heart beats, your lungs take in a breath, and your body temperature increases when you enter a cold room. But your basal metabolic rate (BMR), the rate at which you burn calories just to stay alive, accounts for 70 percent of the calories you burn in a day. (You burn the rest by moving around and by digesting food.)

Not all metabolisms are created equal. Some experts think that your BMR may speed up or slow down in an attempt to maintain a set body weight. So if you overeat, your metabolism burns more calories than usual, even while you are sleeping. If you diet, on the other hand, your body burns fewer calories. For some people, this means that their bodies stay slender no matter how much they eat. For others, it means that their bodies cling to a heavier weight no matter how little they eat.

Genes cast at least 25 percent of the votes and maybe as much as 75 percent, influencing your hormones, the amount of muscle tone you have, and how much and what you eat. Your BMR is not set in stone, however. Your environment, including which foods you choose and how much you restrain your caloric intake, also has an impact. Here is what you can do.

Spice up your life. Eating spicy food may boost your metabolism for 3 hours afterward. In one study, people revved up their calorie-burning potential by 25 percent when they ate food with hot mustard and chili sauce. You don't want to make every meal spicy, however. "It seems that if you eat spices regularly, it may blunt the effect," says Jeya

Henry, Ph.D., professor of biological and molecular science at Oxford Brookes University in Oxford, England. Eating spicy food two to three times a week seems to produce the most benefits.

Eat breakfast. You may plan to eat lunch, but your body doesn't know that. If you skip breakfast, all your body knows is that its food supply has been interrupted, maybe for a long, long time. So it starts burning calories more slowly to keep you from starving during an impending famine. To reassure your metabolism that there's plenty of food to be had and to keep it purring along, eat something when you wake up.

Pick carbohydrates and pass up the fat. Your body burns energy while digesting all kinds of foods. But it may burn more calories in the process of digesting complex carbohydrates than it burns while digesting protein or fat. Make sure you get no more than 25 to 30 percent of your calories from fat and no more than 15 percent from protein foods, such as meats, fish, poultry, and cheese. Get the rest from complex carbohydrates, such as fruits, vegetables, whole wheat pasta, breads, and rice.

Lift your weight. The speed of your resting metabolism is also affected by your muscle mass. The more muscle you have, the faster your metabolic rate. In fact, those who build muscle through weight lifting must eat 15 percent more just to maintain their weight, says Maria A. Fiatarone Singh, M.D., associate professor in the School of Nutrition Science and Policy and chief of the human nutrition and exercise physiology laboratory at the Jean Mayer USDA Human Nutrition Research Center on Aging, both at Tufts University in Boston.

Your Perfect Weight

Are you in love with the wrong weight?

You may have picked your perfect weight at some point when you were young. Or maybe you didn't think about your perfect weight until the day you saw the body you'd love to have but didn't—yet. Although you were satisfied with the way you looked, you knew that if you dropped 10 pounds or so, you, too, could look like that.

Or you may have arrived at your perfect weight with the best of intentions, based simply on what the chart in the doctor's office says is the best weight for you and your health. In any case, the problem is that you can't make it happen.

If your quest for your perfect weight is constantly frustrating you, it may be time to perfect reality. Picking a weight that you want to be but can never attain is self-defeating.

"There's a very large range of healthy weights, and you have to put that range in perspective," says Joanne Curran-Celentano, R.D., Ph.D., associate professor of nutritional sciences at the University of New Hampshire in Durham. "If it's completely stressful for you to keep your

Those Stubborn Pounds

Is it a cruel joke of nature that you can lose 10 pounds in 2 weeks, but you can't shed those last 2 pounds in 10 weeks? Not exactly. Those first 10 pounds were probably mostly water that you lost following a very low calorie, low-carbohydrate diet. When you cut your calories severely, your body draws first on its carbohydrate reserves. When they're gone, your body turns to fat for fuel, a process that releases excess water through your urine. The loss isn't permanent. Here's why.

After a couple of weeks, your body adjusts to your strict diet and starts to conserve energy by lowering its basal metabolic rate (BMR), the rate at which you burn calories just to stay alive. Long periods of calorie restriction can cause your BMR to fall 20 to 30 percent below normal levels. At this point, your body actually requires fewer calories than it previously needed to stay alive and

weight at one number, I don't think it's worth it. I see people spend a whole lot of anxiety and a whole lot of energy trying to maintain a weight that they think is in the appropriate range. They would be a lot freer if they would forget about that weight and concentrate on developing a healthy lifestyle."

In addition to causing anxiety and stress, picking a number that's too low on the scale sets you up for failure, says Susan Olson, Ph.D., a clinical psychologist and weight-management consultant in Seattle and coauthor of *Keeping It Off: Winning at Weight Loss.* The weight-loss process feels excruciating. No matter what the scale tells you, even if it says you've lost weight, you still are not satisfied. You get discouraged, overeat, and gain weight.

healthy. This explains the infamous weight-loss plateau, according to Bernestine B. McGee, R.D., Ph.D., professor and chair of the department of human nutrition and food at Southern University in Baton Rouge, Louisiana.

There is something you can do, however, to burn off those last few pounds: exercise. Exercise helps keep your BMR humming along. Better yet, combine exercise with a sensible eating program, and you'll actually increase your BMR.

Since exercise increases muscle mass, the scale may not be the best indicator of how successful your diet has been. Muscle weighs more than fat. So even though you may be losing fat as you diet and exercise, you may not be losing pounds. For this reason, avoid focusing on the numbers on your scale: instead of wrestling with your weight, just fight fat.

Is Your Weight a Health Risk?

If you are obese—that is, if you are 20 percent over the recommended weight for your height—your primary goal in losing weight should be to improve your health. But here's the surprise: You don't have to get down to "normal" to benefit.

Overweight and obesity have been associated with high blood pressure, high cholesterol, heart disease, gallbladder disease, diabetes, and cancer. You don't have to figure out how far above normal weight you are to know if you are at risk. Just look at your naked body in the mirror, says Joan Marie Conway, Ph.D., research chemist at the USDA Human Nutrition Research Center in Beltsville, Maryland. If you see that you can pinch more than an inch in a few places, you're probably overweight and at risk.

Losing just 10 percent of your body weight can make a big difference in your health risk, says Dr. Curran-Celentano. The best way to do this is to aim to take off no more than a pound a week. For instance, if you weigh 170 pounds, you need to lose only 17 pounds over a period of 17 weeks to significantly improve your health. If you attain that goal and find that you still want to lose, you can aim for another 10 percent.

"Even very modest losses—5 to 10 pounds—can have a significant, positive impact on health," notes Susan Zelitch Yanovski, M.D., obesity expert with the National Institute of Diabetes and Digestive and Kidney Diseases at the National Institutes of Health.

Reach for a "Look"

Most of us think of health as a secondary reason for wanting to lose weight. Looking good is the primary goal. This is where unrealistic expectations start, as in "I could stand to lose 20 pounds. Thirty pounds would be even better." Is it possible, though, that in reality what you could really stand to lose is more like 10 to 15 pounds?

If you're going to set a weight-loss goal, make sure you pick a weight that you can reach and maintain, advises Dr. Curran-Celentano. Pick a number that takes into account not only how slim you want to look but also how slim your body will allow you to look. To find that natural weight, follow this two-step process.

1. Start small. If your weight-loss goal is large, start with the 10 or so pounds you should lose to improve your health. This is the weight you *need* to lose, says Dr. Curran-Celentano.

2. Work toward a number you can live with. When trying to lose pounds, many people aim at something that may not be practical, such as their lowest weights as adults. It is much more realistic and attainable to shoot for a weight you can maintain comfortably for years to come—one that fits your lifestyle.

To determine your best weight, think about a weight that seemed natural for you as an adult. Perhaps you weighed 140 pounds for many years, then suddenly began putting on additional pounds. Take that figure and add a couple of pounds to it. This is your goal weight. It may be somewhat lighter than your healthy weight and somewhat heavier than your desired weight, says Dr. Curran-Celentano, but it is something you can maintain without torturing yourself.

Figuring out your perfect weight means balancing your desires, your needs, your lifestyle, and your body's natural tendencies. "There's no magic number," says Shiriki Kumanyika, R.D., Ph.D., professor and head of the department of human nutrition and dietetics at the University of Illinois at Chicago and a member of the advisory committee that established the U.S. government's 1995 Dietary Guidelines for Americans. "You cannot pick a goal weight off a chart. You have to factor in your own current weight and weight history, your family's health history, your personal health goals, your own eating patterns, and your level of activity. Then you can pick a weight-reduction target that makes sense."

Making Sense
of Weights and Measures

For most of us, weight loss is a numbers game: your weight, your measurements, your percentage of body fat, the number of calories you put in your mouth each day, how many grams of fat you swallow, the serving sizes of foods you eat, and the number of calories you burn.

When it comes to measuring your progress on a weight-loss program, some numbers are more important than others. And plenty of them are downright unnecessary. To find out which numbers we should pay attention to in planning a weight-loss program, we asked nutrition expert Maria A. Fiatarone Singh, M.D., associate professor in the School of Nutrition Science and Policy and chief of the human nutrition and exercise physiology laboratory at the Jean Mayer USDA Human Nutrition Research Center on Aging, both at Tufts University in Boston. Here is her advice.

Chart Your Weight-Loss Course

The basic measurement that we use to decide if we need to lose weight is the number on the scale. We can determine what we need to lose in two ways: the traditional height/weight/body-frame table that you find in your doctor's office or the newer body mass index (BMI), which has been getting a lot of attention for the past few years.

The numbers game: Body mass index (BMI)

The theory: It's more complicated than the insurance table, but it's believed to be a more accurate gauge of what you should weigh. Your BMI is a ratio of height to weight that is an indication of your weight-related health risk. Once you do the calculations, you'll end up with a number between 19 and 32; the closer your BMI is to 19, the better.

How to measure: To find your BMI, you'll need a calculator. Take your height in inches and square it (multiply it by itself). Divide your weight in pounds by that number. Multiply the result by 705.

Here's an example: Let's say you are 5 feet 6 inches and weigh 148 pounds. Your height (66 inches) squared equals 4,356. Divide your weight (148) by 4,356, then multiply the answer by 705. You'll get a BMI of 23.9.

A BMI between 18.5 and 24.9 is considered normal. A BMI between 25.0 and 29.9 means that you are overweight and may be at risk for weight-related disease. Since some women who have BMIs over 25 are perfectly healthy, however, you should take into account other risk factors, such as your family history, eating habits, age, and level of physical activity, before you get alarmed at your number. A BMI of 30 or above means that you are obese and at substantially increased risk for disease.

Strengths: Measuring your BMI goes a step beyond simply stepping onto the scale. It's probably the most accurate and scientific way to predict whether your weight could cause you to die prematurely from cancer, heart disease, or some other weight-related illness. BMI has been used in longevity studies that showed that those under 30 years of age with BMIs of 19 to 22 had the greatest chance of living the longest.

Weaknesses: Many of us want to shoot for one number in particular, but the BMI scale does not allow for such specificity. The difference in health risk between BMIs of 23 and 24, for instance, is minimal. BMI exists purely as a measurement of health risk.

Recommendation: Calculate your BMI at the beginning of a weight-loss plan to find out if you fall into the at-risk category. If your BMI is 30 or higher, you'll want to lower it. Once you start your weight-loss plan, continue to calculate your BMI once a month until you get your result below 30. Once you're there, you don't need to spend a lot of time worrying about your BMI.

The long and the short of it is that those who are lean throughout life or whose weights don't fluctuate greatly from year to year are more likely to lead long, healthy lives. Nevertheless, if you are overweight and lose extra pounds, you can still reduce your risk of osteoarthritis, high blood pressure, diabetes, and other problems.

Weight and Measurements

In recent years, research has found that where we wear our body fat has an impact on factors that are more crucial than beauty. Our body shape is an indicator of our propensity for certain diseases. If you need motivation to lose weight, you might want to get out the tape measure. But there are different ways to interpret what your measurements are saying. Here's the rundown.

The numbers game: Your measurements

The theory: Strategically measuring your waist, hips, and chest or bust can give you an accurate idea of exactly how much smaller your body is getting, helping to motivate you as you fight fat.

Strengths: Measuring your body circumference is much more accurate than stepping on the scale because muscle weighs more than fat. If you build muscle through exercise, you may not lose much weight, according to the scale. Thankfully, however, muscle is also more compact than fat, so your body size will still shrink as you lose fat and gain muscle. And that's where using a tape measure comes in. It lets you know exactly how much smaller you are.

Weaknesses: Too much emphasis can be placed on specific body measurements.

Recommendation: Go for it. Concentrate on your waist size, which will shrink as your belly gets smaller, and your hip circumference, which will provide a good idea of how your rear end and thighs are shaping up.

The numbers game: Waist-to-hip ratio

The theory: Research has shown that your body *shape* may be more important than your body *size* when it comes to assessing weight-related health risks. The fat most associated with health risks makes you look like an apple. It can be found on the upper body, in the abdomen and above, rather than on the thighs and hips. So if your waist is much wider than your hips, you have too much of the more dangerous, upper-body fat.

How to measure: Use a measuring tape to measure your waist at its narrowest point. Then measure your hips at their widest point. Divide your waist measurement by your hip measurement. Anything above 0.85 means that you are more prone to heart disease, high blood pressure, stroke, diabetes, and some types of cancer.

Strengths: Finding the ratio between the measurements of your waist and hips can give you an extremely accurate prediction of whether you will develop life-threatening diseases later in life. Looking at where your fat is distributed also takes genetic influences and lifestyle into

Overnight Weight Gain?

Ever wonder why the scale says you've gained 5 pounds the day after a big pig out? Can you really gain weight overnight?

Of course not. It would take 3,500 *extra* calories to account for just 1 pound gained. And just as your weight can fluctuate from day to day, it can vary throughout the day. One volunteer recorded seven different weights in the course of a day, going from 118.5 pounds right after waking and wearing only underwear to 126.5 pounds right after lunch when fully clothed and with a full bladder.

But if fat is not tipping the scale, what is? Water, for one thing. When you store carbohydrates, they're stored with water, and you can carry a lot of water weight because there are many places to store excess water in your body. If your binge included a lot of salty foods, such as

account. Certain lifestyles, such as eating a high-fat diet and smoking, tend to make fat accumulate in the belly area. On the other hand, both aerobic exercise and resistance training as well as estrogen replacement therapy have been shown to reduce belly fat.

Weaknesses: Although calculating your waist-to-hip ratio is the best method of assessing the health risks of your body shape, your measurements do not tell you how much fat you carry overall. And body measurements don't distinguish well between fat and muscle. So while measurements accurately predict how your body shape affects your health, they don't reflect your level of fitness.

Recommendation: Your waist and hip measurements, rather than your waist-to-hip ratio, are probably the most important numbers game of all.

potato chips, you will retain even more water, making the scales register even more extra pounds.

Unlike fat weight, water weight is transient. If you weighed yourself four more times the next day, the scale would probably say something different every time. In other words, you can turn around a night of overeating by making a few adjustments the next day. The key is to not become discouraged. Try to increase your activity. You may also want to eat some high-fiber foods to avoid constipation.

Finally, if you did eat a lot of salty foods the night before and you're retaining water, believe it or not, the thing to do is drink six to eight glasses of water. This will help you flush out the sodium, which is what's holding the water in.

Expert consulted: Michele Trankina, Ph.D., nutritional physiologist and professor of biological sciences, St. Mary's University, San Antonio

Food Math

When we're not weighing and measuring our bodies, we turn our attention to food. Here is what's worth counting and what's not.

The numbers game: Grams of fat

The theory: Eating fat is more fattening than eating carbohydrate or protein. For one thing, fat has 9 calories per gram, compared with 4 calories per gram for both carbohydrate and protein. Also, fat is stored in fat cells more efficiently than carbohydrate or protein. The body burns off just 3 percent of its fat calories in the process of storing fat. While converting carbohydrate into fat to be stored, however, the body burns 23 percent of the carbohydrate calories. So limiting your fat intake can help you lose weight, regardless of how well you watch your calories.

How to count: Restrict the amount of fat you eat based on your goal weight and your average calorie intake, limiting your fat calories to 25 percent of your daily calorie consumption. For example, if your total daily intake is 1,600 calories, you should be getting no more than 400 calories from fat (and that's equivalent to 44 grams of fat).

Strengths: Counting how many grams of fat you eat in a day is an extremely accurate way of knowing whether you are sticking with your new eating plan.

Weaknesses: Counting is difficult. To succeed, you would have to walk around with a fat-counting guide and a set of measuring cups and spoons. Every time you went out to eat, you'd have to find out exactly how the food was prepared and the size of the portions. And you'd have to write down everything you ate so you could tally it all up at the end of the day.

Recommendation: Don't you have better things to do? Concentrate on slowly cutting fat from your diet. One way to do this is to eat more low-fat whole grains, fruits, and vegetables. These foods fill you up. What's more, by substituting them for higher-fat foods, you automatically reduce calories. You'll find numerous other tips in this book to help you do just that. Every once in a while, you can tally up how much fat you are eating to ensure that you are on target. But don't miss out on more enjoyable ways of spending life by busying yourself with fat-gram counts.

The numbers game: Counting calories

The theory: It's pretty basic. Based on the proven scientific formula that a pound of stored body fat equals 3,500 calories, you should lose a pound for every 3,500 calories you save. So if it takes 2,000 calories a day to maintain your current weight and you go on a 1,500-calorie-a-day diet, you should lose a pound a week.

How to count: Determine the number of calories that your body requires to maintain your current weight. You can do this by measuring and writing down everything you eat for 2 weeks. Use food labels or a calorie-counting guide to figure out how many calories are in the food you eat. At the end of 2 weeks, add it all up and divide by 14. The result is the average number of calories that you are eating each day to maintain your weight. Based on this number, determine how many calories you want to cut every day. For this method to work, you have to count your calories daily.

To lose 1 pound a week, cut 500 calories a day. To lose a ½-pound a week, cut 250 calories a day.

Strengths: As with counting grams of fat, counting calories is an extremely accurate way of knowing whether you are sticking to your eating plan. And eventually, if you can maintain your calorie restriction, you can lose weight.

Weaknesses: If you've ever tried it, you know that no matter how much you stick with the calorie-counting program, you're not necessarily going to drop the weight according to plan, especially if you use the scale as an indicator. As mentioned above, a lot of other factors need to be considered when stepping on the scale. Also, scientists have discovered that our calorie burner has a way of slowing down when we start to conserve calories. For successful weight loss, you need more than calorie control: You need to exercise as well. In addition, counting calories is even more tedious than counting grams of fat, so this whole method can become discouraging and self-defeating.

Recommendation: Forget about it. You can keep up the calorie-counting regimen for a month or two at best, but not for the lifetime it takes to keep weight off.

The numbers game: Tallying calories burned through exercise

The theory: You can boost the number of calories you burn every day by boosting your energy consumption through exercise. The theory holds that exercise also stokes your metabolism so you burn calories more efficiently all day long. However, you have to build calorie-hungry muscle with weight lifting as well as get in a ½ hour or more of heart-pumping aerobic exercise on most days to get the effect.

How to count: To be honest, it's really hard to gauge this accurately because so much depends on your level of fitness. There is a general rule of thumb, however, for how many calories you can expect to burn for any activity. One mile is equal to 100 calories, for example, no matter how long it takes you to cover the distance.

A few other examples are mild walking, 92 calories burned per ½ hour; slow walking, 122 calories; low-impact aerobic dance, 137 calories; weight lifting, 150 calories; swimming, 270 calories; vigorous walking, 277 calories; jogging, 327 calories.

Strengths: Figuring out approximately how many calories you burn during exercise is not quite as difficult as figuring out how many calories you eat. That's about it.

Weaknesses: As we said, it's pretty hard to be accurate about this. Most people exercise moderately, as they should. The truth is, though, that at a moderate pace, you really don't get much of a difference in calorie burning no matter what type of exercise you do, even though various calorie-burning charts indicate otherwise.

Recommendation: Exercise. But don't pick your exercise, time, or intensity based on the number of calories you want to burn. Once you make exercise contingent on how many calories you have to burn, you're more likely to quit. Rather, think of exercise as something that helps you lose weight not merely by burning a certain number of calories per session but also by increasing your metabolic rate, increasing how fast your body burns off calories from food you consume, and helping you to be more active and fit.

The numbers game: Food groups

The theory: Some foods are healthier than others. If you concentrate on making sure that you eat enough of the healthy foods each day, you'll automatically eat fewer of the fattening, unhealthy ones. You'll simply be too full on low-fat, fibrous food to fit in many high-calorie, fat-laden treats. The outcome is that you'll lose weight naturally.

How to count: Each day, try to eat two or three servings of low-fat dairy products, three or four servings of fruit, four servings of vegetables, eight servings of whole grains, and five servings of lean meats and other protein foods, says Joanne Curran-Celentano, R.D., Ph.D., associate professor of nutritional sciences at the University of New Hampshire in Durham. Here's a rough idea of what counts as a serving in each of the food groups.

- Dairy: A cup of milk or yogurt or 1½ ounces of nonfat or low-fat cheese
- Fruit: A medium apple, banana, or orange; ½ cup of chopped cooked or canned fruit; or ¾ cup of fruit juice
- Vegetables: A cup of raw leafy vegetables; ½ cup of other vegetables (cooked or chopped raw); or ¾ cup of vegetable juice
- Grains: One-half bagel; one slice of bread; ¾ cup of ready-to-eat cereal; ½ cup of cooked cereal, rice, or pasta; or 3 cups of popcorn
- Protein: One ounce of cooked lean meat, poultry, or fish; one egg; ½ cup of cooked legumes; 3 ounces of tofu; or 2 tablespoons of peanut butter

Strengths: Keeping track of the types of food you eat throughout the day is much easier and more practical than counting calories or grams of fat. When you eat a banana, for instance, you know you've had one fruit serving. You don't have to weigh it and then look up its calorie or fat content in a book. Because you are dealing with smaller numbers, you can mentally add up what you eat, rather than keep a detailed food diary.

Weaknesses: This method doesn't take into account fruit, vegetable, and grain dishes that are also high in fat and calories, such as eggplant Parmesan, pizza, and fried zucchini. It also doesn't take body size into consideration.

Recommendation: Of all the counting methods, this one works the best. It's the easiest to stick with as well as the most satisfying. You can count food groups for the rest of your life and never feel deprived.

PART TWO

Food and You

Get a Handle on Your Appetite Triggers

Have you ever joked that just the sight of food makes you fat? Or that you can gain weight just by smelling food? To some extent, it's true.

For many, eating behavior is motivated more by external influences, such as the sight and smell of food, than by hunger, says Beverly Cowart, Ph.D., director of the taste and smell clinic at the Monell Chemical Senses Center in Philadelphia. "For some people, it's very difficult not to eat when around food that is very appealing."

Other than what you see or smell, a host of situations inside your body can also arouse your appetite—a surge of the hormone insulin, the release of specific appetite-sensitive chemicals in your brain, or an empty stomach.

Hunger Patrol

Your stomach, brain chemicals known as neurotransmitters, and hormones are prudent, often signaling you to eat only when nutrients are low, urging you to eat when and what you really need to. Your eyes, nose, and tastebuds are more apt to lead you astray. Here's how to train your brain and stomach to be your hunger patrol.

Smell your food. Studies have shown that once you

Q & A

Can Eating Make You Hungry?

Believe it or not, yes. Many people who skip breakfast, for example, say that if they eat in the morning, they're hungrier by lunchtime. Those hunger pangs are a signal that your metabolism is working as it should. So, yes, eating regularly means that you're going to feel hungry regularly, but that's a good thing.

Actually, it's appetite, not hunger, that makes you overeat. Hunger is easy to appease; a little food will take care of it. Appetite is not. What sometimes happens, especially if you're constantly denying your hunger, is that taking the first bite releases your inhibitions. Then it's easy to think, "Now that I'm eating, I might as well keep eating." Hunger is alleviated quickly, but you don't know it because your appetite takes over. You keep on eating.

The best way to deal with hunger is to give in to it. Satisfy your hunger with something small (like carrots) so you keep your metabolism steady. To avoid overeating, pay attention to your body's natural hunger cues. Eat when your stomach tells you to, and stop eating as soon as the pangs go away.

Expert consulted: Joanne Curran-Celentano, R.D., Ph.D., associate professor of nutritional sciences, University of New Hampshire, Durham

start eating, smelling food can make you stop eating sooner by satisfying you faster. So eat more slowly and take the time to smell the food you are eating, says Susan Schiffman, Ph.D., professor of medical psychology in the department of psychiatry at Duke University Medical School in Durham, North Carolina.

Keep a food diary. "Write down any unplanned eating and the circumstances under which it occurred," says Ronette Kolotkin, Ph.D., director of the behavioral program at the Duke University Diet and Fitness Center and coauthor of *The Duke University Medical Center Book of Diet and Fitness*. Review your notes so that you can anticipate appetite triggers and plan to deal with them.

Eat breakfast. Researchers at Vanderbilt University in Nashville put 52 overweight women on a 12-week diet during which some ate three meals a day, including breakfast, while others passed up their morning meal. The women who ate breakfast tended to snack less on high-fat, high-calorie goodies.

Spice it right. Food will satisfy you more quickly if it tastes good and has good mouth feel. One way to guarantee flavor without resorting to large amounts of sugar, salt, or fat is to use plenty of herbal seasonings or other flavorings that tend to be hot or sour, says Dr. Cowart. Think lemon juice, jalapeño peppers, and chili powder.

Eat bargain foods. On a calorie-for-calorie basis, some foods fill you up faster and satisfy your hunger better than others. The faster a food fills you up, the less of it you eat. Examples of filling foods are apples, oranges, potatoes, whole wheat pasta, fish, lean beefsteak, and popcorn.

Don't overdo fat. High-fat meals at any time of the day seem to induce cravings for yet more fat, says Sarah Leibowitz, Ph.D., behavioral neurobiologist at Rockefeller University in New York City. She found that lab rats eating meals that were more than 40 percent fat continued to produce high levels of a neurochemical that stimulates an appetite for fat.

A study by researchers at England's University of Leeds suggests this also holds true for human appetite-control

What Are Your Appetite Triggers?

To determine how much influence different social and emotional triggers have on your eating habits, rate how much influence you think they have, says Susan Head, Ph.D., clinical psychologist at the Duke University Diet and Fitness Center in Durham, North Carolina. To do so, take the following quiz, developed by Shirley M. Glynn, Ph.D., and Audrey J. Ruderman, Ph.D., at the University of Illinois at Chicago. It's given to people who go to the Duke center to lose weight.

For each of the following scenarios, answer the question "How difficult is it to control overeating?" by rating yourself on a scale of one to seven. A rating of one means that you have no difficulty controlling your eating, while a rating of seven means that you can't control it.

1. After work or school _____
2. During the holidays _____
3. When you're with friends _____
4. When you're preparing food _____
5. When you're at a social occasion that centers around food, such as a dinner party _____
6. When you're with family members _____
7. When you feel like sitting back and enjoying food _____
8. When you're faced with tempting food _____
9. When the refrigerator is full _____
10. When you're hungry _____
11. When you feel restless _____

systems. A high-fat meal, it seems, simply isn't as satisfying as a high-carbohydrate meal.

Darken your eating environment. Bright colors like orange, red, and yellow stimulate the appetite far more than

12. When you feel upset _____
13. When you feel tense _____
14. When you feel irritable _____
15. When you're annoyed _____
16. When you're angry at someone _____
17. When you're angry with yourself _____
18. When you're depressed _____
19. When you feel impatient _____
20. After an argument _____
21. When you feel frustrated _____
22. When you want to cheer up _____
23. When you feel overly sensitive _____
24. When you're nervous _____
25. When you're anxious or worried _____

Add up your ratings for all 25 scenarios to get your score. A score between 54 and 106 is average and means you are fairly confident you can handle various appetite triggers. The lower your score, the less likely you are to eat in response to appetite triggers. A higher score means many situations cause you to overeat. Now look over the quiz to isolate your worst appetite triggers.

Scenarios 1 through 10 deal with social situations, while 11 through 25 deal with emotional triggers. If your answers for the first 10 add up to less than 35, you have a good handle on how you eat in social situations. If your answers for 11 through 25 add up to less than 50, you deal effectively with emotional triggers.

dark ones like gray, black, and brown, says Maria Simonson, Sc.D., Ph.D., professor emeritus and director of the health, weight, and stress clinic at the Johns Hopkins Medical Institutions in Baltimore. So a dark tablecloth and napkins can tame your appetite tiger.

Avoid the buffet table. "The variety and presentation of good-tasting, calorie-rich foods that are often found on buffet tables can be too tempting," says Dr. Kolotkin.

Tune in to some slow mood music. People chew faster and eat more to spirited tunes than to slow, restful ones, according to Dr. Simonson. So Bach may be a better dinner companion than Bruce Springsteen.

Watch for crowded encounters. Researchers at Georgia State University in Atlanta have found that we all eat more when we dine with company. When dining in large groups, in fact, we tend to eat about 75 percent more than when dining alone.

Get more exercise. "Exercise can decrease the appetite," says Dr. Simonson. A 20- to 60-minute workout three to five times a week should do it.

Play with your food. "When you go to a restaurant, order food that has lots of potential to keep your hands busy and that will take longer to eat—hot soup, for example, or lobster in the shell," recommends Angie Day, former executive director of the Phoenix Spa in Houston.

Wear something tight-fitting when you go out to eat. "Being a little uncomfortable is a nice little reminder that you're trying to lose weight, and it will keep you from overeating," says Day. "It's a trick that works for me."

Think, Don't Shovel

To short-circuit automatic-pilot eating, go through the following four-step process at mealtime.

1. Two minutes before the meal: Sit quietly in your chair. Take five or six long, deep breaths. Let yourself feel relaxed.

2. One minute before the meal: Think about the work that was required to prepare and cook the food. Appreciate the fact that it's going into your body to nourish you.

3. Midway through the meal: Take another minute. Stop eating, and take five deep breaths. Sit quietly for just a moment. You might even realize that you're not hungry anymore.

4. Ten minutes after eating: Take 1 minute to do another series of five deep breaths. Focus on the physical sensations that the food might be causing in your body. Hopefully, most are pleasant.

Cravings, Go Away!

High-fat food makes a high-fat body. Ounce for ounce, dietary fat has more than twice the calories of and is more readily converted into body fat than either protein or carbohydrate. So cutting your fat intake way back is a crucial element in an effective weight-control plan.

How much fat is optimal? You've probably heard that 30 percent of calories from fat should be your goal, but this recommendation is based more on healthy living and disease prevention than on weight loss. Some experts recommend 10 percent, but that's too strict and too hard to follow. Instead, aim for 25 percent.

Fortunately, carving fat from your diet is not difficult. In fact, once you start eating less fat, you'll feel full more often. That's because low-fat food has fewer calories. You'll be able to eat more and still lose weight.

Many people also report that fatty foods start to lose their appeal the longer low-fat diets continue. In one 4-year study, for example, more than 2,000 participants who limited their fat intake to around 25 percent of calories lost their taste for fat within 6 months or less. By the end of the study, many said they honestly didn't like fatty foods anymore.

So how do you go from loving fatty foods to snubbing them?

Cutting Back Made Easy

At first, holding your fat intake to 25 percent of calories will seem tedious. That's because counting your daily grams of fat, at least for a little while, is the best way to learn how to eyeball your fat intake. For a couple of weeks, keep track of the food you eat, says Marsha Hudnall, R.D., director of nutrition programs at Green Mountain at Fox Run, a health and weight-management community for women in Ludlow, Vermont. Packaged foods have labels that tell the number of calories and grams of fat per serving. For nonpackaged foods, consult a calorie and fat-gram guide, available at most bookstores and libraries.

For each day, add up the number of calories and grams of fat you eat. Remember, one gram of fat has 9 calories, so if you eat 1,600 calories, limit yourself to about 44 grams of fat a day to stay within the guidelines, says Hudnall.

Once you get an idea of how much fat you are eating, you can take a look at the types of foods you wrote down and look for ways to siphon off fat. All animal foods have fat, so you'll want to start there. That doesn't mean you have to cut them out of your diet, but you can make quick fat savings simply by choosing fat-free milk over whole, buying low-fat cheeses, and opting for leaner meats such as chicken and turkey.

Making the switch to low-fat, however, doesn't mean that you must give up your high-fat favorites. You can still have the foods you love as long as you pay attention to portion sizes and learn how to cut fat without compromising taste. Here are some expert strategies.

Redesign your plate. If you put the average American meal on one of those paper plates with dividers, the largest section—about half of the plate—is filled with meat. The

---

Q & A

Why Can't I Stop at One Potato Chip?

Many people have a love affair with fat and salt and things that crunch. Chips' combination of all three makes them a prime candidate for food addiction.

Studies have shown that if you swear off salt and fat, your cravings for foods like potato chips will increase for the first 3 months. But if you can manage to hold out for 5 months, you'll barely be able to stand the stuff.

A recent trend in snack foods, however, just may be your savior. Crunch is finding its way into a variety of low-fat foods. While crunch may have appeal in part because it's often found in high-fat snacks like chips, it has a stellar reputation of its own for satisfying all kinds of appetites. Crunch is associated with fun and freshness. In some cases, eating crunchy foods can also relieve stress.

One way to avoid eating too many salty, greasy chips, then, is to substitute lighter, lower-fat crunchies, especially baked chips and crackers that taste pretty similar to the originals. Of course, you don't want to get in too deep with those crispy goodies. It's easy to get carried away, even with low-fat, low-salt alternatives.

Expert consulted: Barbara Levine, R.D., Ph.D., director of the nutrition information center, Cornell University Medical College, New York City

rest contains refined starchy food and fat. The meal ends up with 34 to 36 percent of its calories from fat. Instead of plopping meat in the large section, move it to one of the smaller areas. When the meat fills no more than one-quarter of the plate, it generally becomes the 3-ounce serving that earns "very healthy" kudos.

Fill the largest section with vegetables, and put grains in the other space, says Lori Wiersema, R.D., associate director of the Johns Hopkins Weight Management Center in Baltimore. "Redesigning your plate to create the right fuel mix automatically slashes fat and calories to a healthy level," she says.

Use fat judiciously. "You can't just leave out the fat completely because fat tastes really good. But you can compensate," says Marie Simmons, author of *Fresh and Fast* and monthly food columnist for the magazine *Bon Appétit.* "If a recipe calls for ¼ cup of olive oil, for instance, use just 1 tablespoon of oil during cooking and then maybe add another ½ tablespoon at the end so you still have that good taste."

Satisfy with less meat. Meat is one of the top fat sources in our diets. A great way to enjoy smaller portions of meat is to give it an intense flavor, says Marilyn C. Majchrzak, R.D., food-development manager at the Canyon Ranch health resort in Tucson.

At Canyon Ranch, for example, culinary experts top broiled fish with a richly flavored sauce of freshly crushed herbs added to a teaspoon of melted butter. And don't forget eye appeal: When it's thinly sliced and artfully arranged, 3 ounces of chicken looks like no paltry poultry.

Think juicy. If you're used to sautéing vegetables in a ½-inch of oil, cook them in a nonstick pan over low heat in a mixture of a little oil plus water, says Simmons.

Be spicier. If you learn to cook with herbs and spices, you won't miss the taste of butter or oil.

Be saucy. To pare fat calories from muffins, cakes, and other home-baked goodies, swap the cooking fat for applesauce. This trick works best in recipes containing liquid ingredients such as fat-free milk or fruit. Merely substitute one part applesauce for one part oil, butter, or margarine. Instead of using ⅓ cup of oil and two whole eggs when preparing lemon cake from a mix, for example, use ⅓ cup of applesauce and three egg whites. You'll save almost 5 grams of fat and 40 calories per slice.

Serve special spuds. You'll never miss fat-drenched french fries if you make delicious, nutrient-rich sweet potato fries. Cut the unpeeled potatoes into thick slices (about ½ inch), then dredge them in a mixture of low-sodium soy sauce and a few drops of sesame oil. Grill or broil until crisp and golden.

Retrain Your Tastebuds

Instead of seeing your entrance into the low-fat world as torture, view it as an adventure, one where you get to try new recipes and taste new foods. That simple change in your mindset can go a long way toward helping your tastebuds adjust to this new way of eating, thus reducing some of those cravings for high-fat foods. Here are some other strategies.

Take baby steps. Instead of shocking your tastebuds by avoiding all of the foods you love the most, take on a smaller battle. For instance, if you're a real meat person, don't go cold turkey. Instead, try going from a stuffed pork chop to a center-cut pork loin medallion, from a full-size steak to a baby filet mignon, or from a chicken drumstick to a breast. "And once a week, have a meatless meal featuring pasta or grains and vegetables or maybe a lentil-and-brown-rice pilaf. Little by little, increase the number

Foods That Stop Cravings

Sometimes, the best thing you can do when you have a craving is to follow the advice of your stomach: "Eat something." You don't, however, have to eat something fattening to satisfy your yearning. Here are some alternatives.

Suck on a pickle. Pickles are a wonderful combination of powerful flavor and almost no calories.

Combine peppermint and fruit. A really strong craving for sweets can often be stifled by eating a peppermint and washing it down with a few ounces of fruit juice or a few nibbles of fruit, such as an apple or pear.

Spike a yogurt. Cinnamon, vanilla, and nutmeg can satisfy a sweet tooth since these spices add a sweet flavor without the calories. Add the flavorings to yogurt or steamed milk.

Sip some soup. Due to its sheer volume, soup takes up more space in your stomach than other foods, but since it's mostly liquid, you feel fuller on fewer calories.

Sniff a banana, a green apple, or peppermint. In one study, people sniffed from inhalers scented with banana, green apple, or peppermint whenever they felt the urge to have something to eat. On average, they lost almost 5 pounds a month, even though they were told not to change their usual eating patterns. Researchers speculate that the smells may have short-circuited their appetites.

of these dishes," says Bernice Veckerelli, chef at the Norwich Inn Spa in Norwich, Connecticut.

Or let's say that you decide to eat less red meat. Keep track of how much you usually eat in a week. If you find that you're eating seven meat meals a week, for example, first cut back to six by substituting a fish or vegetarian meal. Then go to five, then four, then three. And don't try to be perfect because it just leads to guilt and frustration and quitting. Instead of zero, aim for three.

Don't get bored. "Eat a variety of foods," says Veckerelli, even if you're having weight-loss success with particular tried-and-true items. "A lot of the time, people think that dieting means nothing but grapefruit or fruit and cottage cheese, and eventually they get bored and hungry," she says. But if you make a point of experimenting at mealtime, particularly trying to increase your intake of whole grains, fruits, and vegetables, which are very filling and satisfying, you'll perk up your palate and be more apt to stick with your weight-loss plan.

Allow for some fat. Remember that you are reining in your fat count to 25 percent of calories, not 15 or 10 or 5 percent. Many people crave high-fat foods because they are overrestricting their fat intakes, says Hudnall. They feel deprived. And usually, they eventually pig out on fried chicken, french fries, and cheesecake. You can cut such intense fat cravings by budgeting for an occasional high-fat food, which will fight deprivation cravings. This is a low-fat diet, not a no-fat diet.

Never say, "Just a taste." These three words can be damning to your diet and your psyche. Chances are, you'll eat more if you keep picking from the bag of chips than you would if you ate a full meal. In other words, those little "tastes" can add up, and you can end up eating more than if you set out to eat a predefined portion. Even worse, your psyche won't be satisfied. "If you're yearning for a particular food, serve yourself a reasonable portion," says Jennifer Stack, R.D., nutritionist at New York University Behavioral Health Programs in New York City. You'll feel freed of your hunger—and your craving—after allowing yourself a snack that's sizable enough to satisfy you.

Walk away from cravings. The kind of craving that kicks in at the sight of an ice cream sandwich may dissipate after 10 to 15 minutes if you get moving, says Maria Simonson, Sc.D., Ph.D., professor emeritus and director of the health, weight, and stress clinic at Johns Hopkins Medical Institutions in Baltimore. So walk around the building a few times while on the way to the vending machine. By the time you get there, the ice cream may have lost its appeal.

Lift weights. Weight lifting may naturally curb your hankering for fat. In a study at Brigham Young University in Provo, Utah, 30 women who did nine common strength-training exercises naturally cut back on their fat intakes within 6 weeks, without anyone's having told them to. Researchers suspect that the positive physical changes brought about by weight lifting gave the women the inspiration they needed to change their diets as well.

Take a small bite out of chocolate cravings. Chocolate cravings are harder to resist than most, says Elizabeth Somer, R.D., nutritionist and author of *Nutrition for Women* and *Food and Mood*. If you can't resist, try getting by with a very small piece of something chocolate. To make sure you have only a little, eat your treat with a meal. When you eat chocolate with a meal, you're less likely to overdo it than if you tackle a jumbo chocolate bar and nothing else. Another strategy: If you must have chocolate, choose baked goods made with low-fat cocoa powder, she says.

Get the lowdown on high-risk situations. "Different people have different vulnerabilities," says Joyce D. Nash, Ph.D., a clinical psychologist in San Francisco and Palo Alto, California, and author of *The New Maximize Your Body Potential*. You might, for instance, do fine at an ice cream stand but lose all control at a buffet table. Someone else might handle buffets like a pro but go to pieces at the sight of Reese's Pieces.

"Ask yourself what your high-risk situations are," says Dr. Nash. "Are they going out with friends, when you're feeling down and sorry for yourself, when you're in a bakery? Do a personal analysis. Once you know your eating triggers, you can focus your efforts and determine which strategies you can use to cope better."

Limit alcohol. Although alcohol itself doesn't have fat, drinking it can make you crave fatty foods, says Cindy Wachtler, R.D., a nutritionist in private practice in Dallas. "If you drink a glass of wine before dinner, suddenly the food looks better and tastes better and your judgment of quantities diminishes," she says.

Nix the fat-free bingeing. "Remember, there are calories in fat-free foods," says Stack. It's better to eat that one full-fat candy bar and satisfy your craving for the day than to load up on twice as many calories by eating foods made with fat facsimiles.

Mini-Meals:
When More Means Less

You would think that skipping meals would result in eating fewer calories, which in turn would result in less body fat. But your body doesn't work that way. It actually burns fat more effectively when you eat small amounts of food more often. In fact, scientists have discovered that eating four to six small meals a day actually helps to speed up your fat-burning system. Here's why.

• If you bypass breakfast and skimp on lunch, you're going to overload at dinner. "After an all-day fast, the body is ravenous, and you end up doubling the quantity of food you eat," says Diane Grabowski-Nepa, R.D., nutrition educator at the Pritikin Longevity Center in Malibu, California. Too much food at any one time is too much for your body to handle, and it encourages fat storage. On top of that, your body is more efficient at storing fat in the evening than earlier in the day, when you're more active. So if you overeat at dinner, more calories get stored as fat than, say, if you overeat at breakfast.

• Skipping meals can slow your metabolism by as much as 5 percent. That's because an empty stomach makes your brain think that your body is starving, so it turns down its calorie-burning thermostat in an effort to live longer off its stored fat. On the other hand, when you eat small meals all day long, your stomach never gets a chance to be empty, thus keeping your metabolism purring along.

• When you eat a big meal such as a huge dinner, your body produces insulin, which prevents fat cells from releasing fat into the bloodstream to be picked up by other tissues and burned. In other words, high insulin levels put a lock on your fat-releasing ability. Higher insulin levels also stimulate appetite, which makes you want to eat more. On the other hand, when you eat small meals all day long, you never experience the insulin surge that larger meals create.

• Your stomach expands and contracts with food load, apparently losing its tone when repeatedly pushed to the max. So once it's overstretched, it takes more food to satisfy you, according to studies by scientists at the obesity research center at St. Luke's–Roosevelt Hospital Center in New York City. Eating small amounts of food all day doesn't stretch your stomach, so you feel full more quickly.

Mini-Meal Magic

Ready to give mini-meals a try? Think variety. You want to continue to eat from all the food groups—grains, fruits, vegetables, dairy, and protein—throughout the day. But you don't need to balance your intake of food groups at every meal as you did when you were eating three meals. Instead, you want to achieve balance over the course of an entire day, which means about eight servings of grains, three or four fruits, four vegetables, two or three dairy products, and five lean meats or other protein foods each day.

Here's the best advice from experts for getting into the mini-meal mindset.

Give your regular meals the split. Try dividing what you eat for breakfast, lunch, and dinner in half to create six meals, suggests Anne Dubner, R.D., a nutrition consultant in private practice in Houston. If you usually eat a bagel for breakfast, for example, eat half when you get up and the other half later. If you have a sandwich for lunch, eat the halves at two different times. That way, you won't spend any more time preparing food.

Watch the fat and the portions. In determining your daily intake, it's important to keep your eye on two different horizons: fat and calories. While fat reduction is the most important priority for good health and weight loss, you don't want calories to fall too low or climb too high.

Eat "fat-fighting" foods. That means foods high in fiber and low in fat and added sugar, which in turn means things like fruits, vegetables, and whole wheat bread. Avoid empty-calorie snacks like doughnuts.

Select a serving. Favor foods that are already portioned into individual servings, like a baked potato, a container of yogurt, or a bagel. Eating a set portion ensures that you'll stop when you're full (or nearly full) because you'll run out of food, says Michele Harvey, R.D., a diabetes educator and private nutrition consultant in Boca Raton and Delray Beach, Florida.

Choose no-risk foods. As you adapt, says Dubner, choose low-calorie foods.

Go to pieces. Mini-meals will be more satisfying if you eat them in small bites, says Dubner. So instead of one big rice cake, have a few of the bite-size variety. Instead of

(continued on page 62)

A Mini-Meal Menu Sampler

It can be a little daunting to figure out how to eat all day and still lose weight, so we asked Anne Dubner, R.D., a nutrition consultant in private practice in Houston, to put together a sampling of daily menus to show how satisfying mini-meals can be.

Day One

Breakfast: Half of a whole wheat bagel with pureed roasted peppers mixed with reduced-fat or fat-free cream cheese, an 8-ounce glass of fat-free milk, and ½ cup of blueberries

Snack: The other half of the bagel with roasted peppers

Lunch: Half of a turkey club sandwich (made with turkey breast, sliced tomato, and lettuce) and a mixed garden salad with 1 tablespoon of reduced-fat Russian dressing

Snack: The other half of the sandwich

Dinner: Two cups of pasta primavera (made with rotini pasta, frozen mixed vegetables, garlic, Parmesan cheese, and 1 tablespoon of olive oil) and a slice of Italian bread topped with 1 teaspoon of reduced-fat margarine mixed with 1 teaspoon each of crushed fresh garlic and grated Parmesan cheese

Snack: An oatmeal raisin cookie

Day Two

Breakfast: One slice of raisin bread with 1 tablespoon of peanut butter and a 4-ounce glass of orange juice

Snack: A reduced-fat fig bar and an 8-ounce glass of fat-free milk

Lunch: Half of a chicken salad pita sandwich (made with low-fat cubed cooked chicken, toasted walnuts, raisins, small grapes, and honey) and 1 cup of raw vegetables such as baby carrots and celery

Snack: The other half of the sandwich

Dinner: Cheese quesadilla (made with a fat-free flour tortilla, 2 tablespoons of shredded reduced-fat Cheddar cheese, 1½ teaspoons of chopped canned green chili peppers, 1½ teaspoons of sliced black olives, salsa, and chili powder) with ½ cup of white rice mixed with 2 tablespoons of salsa

Snack: Eight ounces of nonfat flavored yogurt with three graham crackers

Day Three

Breakfast: An English muffin with scrambled egg substitute, an orange wedge, and an 8-ounce glass of fat-free milk

Snack: A sandwich made with half of a banana and 1 tablespoon of peanut butter

Lunch: A small Greek salad (made with chopped tomatoes, cucumbers, sweet red peppers, and onions, with feta cheese and a dressing of lemon juice and olive oil with oregano and garlic) and a slice of Italian bread

Snack: Six crackers with tuna salad (made with tuna, 1 tablespoon of reduced-fat mayonnaise, and a squirt of lemon juice)

Dinner: Potato skins (made with one quartered baked potato, 1 cup of shredded reduced-fat Cheddar cheese, some scallions or chives, and paprika) with ½ cup of steamed broccoli

Snack: Three cups of reduced-fat popcorn sprinkled with 2 teaspoons of Parmesan cheese

eating a big pretzel, have lots of small ones. You can even cut a cookie into pieces and eat the pieces individually.

Don't tempt yourself. If you know that you have no resistance to certain foods—like cookies, for instance—stay away from them. If you don't, you'll probably end up eating well beyond fullness. Choose mini-meal foods that you know you can control, says Donna Weihofen, R.D., nutritionist at the University of Wisconsin Hospital and Clinics in Madison.

Watch out for fat-free. Most packaged fat-free foods won't fill you up for very long. Also, many fat-free foods have added sugar to make up for the loss of fat, points out Weihofen.

Be a Time Machine

Eating mini-meals doesn't have to be time-consuming, according to Natalie Payne, R.D., nutritionist at the Washington Cancer Institute and Washington Hospital Center in Washington, D.C. Here are some timesaving strategies.

Take mini-meals on the road. Keep a snack stash in your car; carry snacks when you go to the mall; and stock your briefcase when you fly. Good portables include small boxes of raisins, mini-boxes of cereal, cans of low-sodium vegetable juice cocktail, and whole wheat hard pretzels.

Switch meals. Consider some easy-to-prepare, easy-to-eat (but somewhat unusual) choices for your meals. Make a turkey sandwich in the evening, for example, and put it in the fridge. Then grab it on your way out the door in the morning and eat it for breakfast on your way to work.

Keep it cold. If you don't have access to a refrigerator where you work, freeze a juice box overnight and put it in the bottom of your lunch bag the following day. The frozen juice will keep cold easy-to-eat items such as yogurt and cheese.

Stash some safe bets. At work, keep a desk drawer stocked with canned fruit (in water or fruit juice), dried fruit, low-fat crackers, and other nonperishable convenience foods. (And don't forget a can opener.)

Slice at night. When slicing up carrots and other raw vegetables for dinner, remember to slice some extras to take along and munch the next day at work.

Dinner: Think Small

Dinner can be the toughest time to eat a mini-meal. If you go out to eat, you're served too much food. If you eat at home, you might linger at the table with the family and eat more than you planned. Here are some ways to think small at dinnertime.

Have an appetizer. Have a snack ready in the fridge for when you walk in the door after work, says Dubner. After you've eaten, change into comfortable clothes, take a shower, or do whatever else you do to ready yourself for an evening meal with your family. Then you can spend as much time at the dinner table as you like, but you won't overeat because you won't be as hungry.

Don't stay on course. Switch back and forth between courses by alternating bites of your main dish (chicken or pasta, for example) with a bite of salad. If you do that, says Dubner, you won't finish eating before the rest of your family does.

Fill 'er up. Before ordering dinner at a restaurant, drink a big glass of water to quiet your appetite, says Dubner. Then take a sip of water after every bite so that you'll eat more slowly.

Hold the bread. When dining out, ask the server not to serve the bread. Or take one roll and send back the basket, says Harvey.

Try a smaller portion. At a restaurant, ask the server for a smaller portion, says Harvey. You can request a meal that's half the usual size, for instance.

Don't entrée right away. When eating out, have a small bowl of noncreamy soup such as minestrone or a small salad before making a decision on your entrée, says Dubner. That way, you won't be as hungry and you'll order a smaller meal.

Or don't order it at all. Instead of ordering an entrée, order an appetizer, says Harvey.

Start low, end high. Eat your vegetables first, then the starches, such as potatoes and bread. Leave the highest-calorie and fattiest items like meat for last, says Dubner. That way, you'll fill up on the lowest-calorie items and feel too full to finish the high-calorie foods.

Take it home. Before the server brings the meal, ask for a doggie bag. Then, when the dinner is served, immediately divide your food in half, putting part in the take-home container and leaving the rest on your plate. Or ask the server to do it for you. Store the take-home container under your chair so you won't be tempted to nibble from it, says Dubner.

Don't worry about detours. Every once in a while—at Thanksgiving, for instance—you'll stuff yourself. Don't feel guilty. If you continually berate yourself, you'll feel so bad about yourself that you'll keep eating.

Breakfasts of Champion Weight Losers

If you skip breakfast, you can shave off 300 to 400 calories and maybe about 10 minutes of preparation and chewing time. But you'll probably eat more, get fatter, and lose time in the long run.

Studies have shown that thin people tend to be breakfast eaters, while overweight people tend to be breakfast skippers. There are plenty of reasons for this. For one, if you don't eat breakfast, you're in for a crash around midmorning. If you're lucky, you'll make it to lunch. Either way, you're likely to overeat or make poor food choices.

"When people skip breakfast, they get tired and irritable," says Bonnie Spring, Ph.D., professor of psychology at Finch University of Health Sciences/Chicago Medical School. "They also experience food cravings. Their hunger may become so intense that they overeat before they feel satisfied. Or they may grab something sugary or fattening in an effort to boost their mood."

So you actually end up making up for and well surpassing the 300 to 400 calories you thought you saved by skipping breakfast. And because you're energy-drained, it takes you longer to get things done, which means you lose more time than the 10 minutes you thought you were saving.

Breakfast skippers also risk slowing their metabolisms. "Breakfast is the day's most important meal because it's your body's signal that it's time to fight fat," says Jan McBarron, M.D., a weight-control specialist and director of Georgia Bariatrics in Columbus. While you sleep, your

---

Q & A

Do I Have to Eat Breakfast?

When you wake up in the morning, your body's fuel level is very low. If you try to get through your busy morning without breakfast, you're running on reserves.

Many people who struggle with their weight skip breakfast and skimp on lunch. By the time they finally do eat, they lose control. But if you eat an adequate breakfast, followed by your usual lunch, you'll be much better off. You won't be ravenously hungry at the end of the day, and you won't feel that you're entitled to a double-size dinner after running on reserves all day.

Even if you're not hungry when you wake up, think of a morning meal as refueling your body. It needn't be a big, heavy meal—have some fruit, cereal and fat-free milk, toast, or a roll.

Another way to help make eating breakfast a habit is to avoid snacking too much late at night, which can leave you feeling full in the morning. Eating at night is like stoking the fire when the demand for fuel is low.

Expert consulted: Abby Bloch, R.D., Ph.D., coordinator of clinical nutrition research, Memorial Sloan-Kettering Hospital, New York City

body stores food as fat so that you have energy to burn when you're awake. Eating lets your fat-burning enzymes know that it's time to get up and go to work. If you don't eat, your body will continue to store fat.

No More Excuses

What are the two most common excuses for skipping breakfast? Number one: Not enough time to make breakfast. Number two: No appetite in the morning. It's time to stop the excuses and do something.

Stop eating at night. Those who tend to skip breakfast also tend to eat the majority of their food late in the day, usually after 6:00 P.M., says Diane Grabowski-Nepa, R.D., nutrition educator at the Pritikin Longevity Center in Malibu, California. Such late-night eating keeps you from being hungry when you wake up. But it also contributes to weight gain because a sleeping body can't burn off the food as quickly as a moving body. Food gets stored as fat instead.

Gradually start eating more in the morning. If you are not hungry in the morning, start gradually. Your first few breakfasts might consist solely of a piece of fruit such as an apple or a banana, says Grabowski-Nepa. "It's better to get something in your system than to go without," she says. Other ideas for small breakfasts include yogurt or an oat bran muffin. Once you get into the habit of eating a small breakfast, move on to more substantial items, like whole wheat bagels.

Go for convenience. Pouring a bowl of cereal and eating it takes less than 10 minutes. Yogurt, oat bran muffins, bagels, and fruit are other good foods that you can eat on the go.

Do other things first. Some people, no matter how little they eat the night before, are not hungry when they first wake up. No problem. Instead of eating breakfast right away, take a shower first. Get dressed, then have breakfast. Or drive to work and then eat. "There's no rule that says you must have breakfast as soon as you roll out of bed," says Grabowski-Nepa. "You can wait for an hour."

You do, however, want to try to eat breakfast within the first couple of hours after waking up.

Be nontraditional. No law forces you to eat traditional breakfast foods for breakfast. "Try beans and rice wrapped in a corn tortilla, which is one of my breakfast favorites,"

The Fat-Fighter's Best Breakfasts

To help you make the best fat-fighting choices at breakfast, Tina Ruggiero, R.D., a nutritionist with The Food Group in New York City, came up with a list of bad, better, and best options. To qualify as a best breakfast, foods had to be low in fat and calories and high in fiber, vitamins, minerals, and other nutrients.

Omelets

Bad: Three-egg cheese omelet served with three strips of bacon and two slices of buttered white toast (700 calories and 48 grams of fat)

Better: Three-egg omelet made with egg substitute and filled with cheese and spinach, served with one strip of bacon and two slices of white toast with low-sugar jam (560 calories and 26 grams of fat)

Best: Three-egg omelet made with egg substitute and filled with 1 ounce of low-fat cheese, ¼ cup of chopped mushrooms, and ½ cup of spinach; served with ½ cup of water-packed fruit salad and one slice of whole wheat toast with 1 tablespoon of low-sugar jam (400 calories and 10 grams of fat) says Grabowski-Nepa. Or consider leftovers or perhaps a turkey sandwich on whole-grain bread. Just make sure it's low in fat.

Blend a breakfast drink. If you really can't stand the thought of eating breakfast, drink it instead. Try a fruity, frosty shake, suggests Judith S. Stern, R.D., Sc.D., professor of nutrition and internal medicine at the University of California at Davis. The night before, slice half of a banana and freeze it. In the morning, toss the sliced banana into a blender with about ½ cup of sliced strawberries and

Pancakes

Bad: Short stack (three) with butter, syrup, and two sausage patties (560 calories and 35 grams of fat)

Better: Short stack with butter, syrup, and two slices of Canadian bacon (430 calories and 19 grams of fat)

Best: Short stack with 1 teaspoon of margarine, 1 tablespoon of reduced-calorie syrup, and fresh peach slices (355 calories and 15 grams of fat)

Sandwiches versus Oatmeal

Bad: Ham, egg, and cheese sandwich; hash browns; and orange juice (600 calories and 27 grams of fat)

Better: English muffin with fat-free cream cheese, hash browns, and orange juice (440 calories and 12 grams of fat)

Best: Hot oatmeal mixed with ½ cup of assorted berries and fat-free milk, served with ⅛ of a honeydew melon and 8 ounces of apricot nectar (440 calories and 2 grams of fat)

a cup of fat-free milk. Add a drop or two of lemon juice to give the shake some extra flavor. If you forget to freeze the banana, you can still blend it, but add an ice cube. You can also try adding peaches and cinnamon instead of strawberries and lemon.

Turn in. One way to help yourself get up early enough to have time for breakfast is to go to bed earlier. Gradually start heading for bed a few minutes earlier than normal. Make no more than 15 minutes of change per week. Then set your alarm so that you get up a little bit earlier every day. You'll know that you have adjusted when you start waking up just before your alarm goes off.

The Best Breakfast

The best breakfasts are also the easiest to prepare. What are the best? Oatmeal and other whole-grain hot cereals are the most filling and satisfying breakfast foods you can eat, says Grabowski-Nepa. "For a lot of people who don't have time, it might seem like too much work," she says. "But you can microwave it. It takes only a couple of minutes."

Running a close fat-fighting second is a low-sugar, high-fiber cold cereal; whole-grain breads come in third.

Here are a few things to keep in mind when choosing breakfast foods.

Think fiber. High-fiber foods such as whole-grain breads, oatmeal, and some cold cereals help to keep your blood sugar levels stable, which in turn helps you avoid cravings later. They also make you feel full faster and longer.

When picking out breakfast cereals, look for ones that have at least 4 grams of fiber per serving, says Grabowski-Nepa. (You can find out by checking the nutrition label on the box.) The more fiber the cereal has, the better. You can get even more fiber by adding some blueberries, a sliced banana, or other fruit to your cereal.

Avoid sugar. "A lot of people eat a real sugary cereal at 8:00 in the morning, and by 9:00 they're ravenous," says Grabowski-Nepa. That's because the high amount of sugar makes the body overproduce insulin, which then signals you to eat more. Look for cereals in which sugar is not the first ingredient listed on the label.

Group your foods. Once you become a bona fide breakfast eater, try to work a few different food groups into your morning routine. Think dairy, complex carbohydrate, and fruit.

To get your dairy, you could have nonfat yogurt, fat-free milk, or nonfat cream cheese or sour cream. Dairy foods give you the protein you need to help sustain your satiety until you eat lunch or a mid-morning snack. For carbohydrate, try hot or cold cereal, whole wheat toast or a bagel, or an oat bran muffin. For fruit, have a banana, blueberries, strawberries, or orange juice.

"People feel more satisfied when they have a variety of foods," says Grabowski-Nepa. "Plus, you eat more nutrients." Here are some energizing multi-food-group breakfast ideas.

- Have a toasted whole wheat bagel with a tablespoon of peanut butter, 8 ounces of fat-free milk, and a banana.
- Try ¾ cup of oatmeal cooked with fat-free milk and topped with 2 tablespoons of wheat germ, 1 tablespoon of honey or brown sugar, 1 tablespoon of chopped nuts, and 1 tablespoon of raisins. Serve with 6 ounces of apple juice.
- Try egg substitute scrambled with green peppers and onions and topped with some salsa. Serve with a fat-free flour tortilla and 6 ounces of orange juice.

Figure on fruit. "Every meal should include a fruit or vegetable," says Cheryl Rock, Ph.D., associate professor of nutrition in the department of family and preventive medicine at the University of California, San Diego, School of Medicine. Breakfast is no exception to this rule. Concentrate on deep yellow fruits like cantaloupe, which provides beta-carotene along with vitamin C. Or try a peach, a mango, ½ cup of berries, a banana, half a grapefruit, or ¼ cup of raisins. Or try 6 ounces of 100 percent orange, cranberry, or strawberry-kiwi juice.

Combine protein with carbohydrate. "If you eat all carbohydrate at a meal, you'll feel sleepy in an hour or so," says Elizabeth Somer, R.D., nutritionist and author of *Nutrition for Women* and *Food and Mood*. A favorite power breakfast of Somer's is quick and easy: a tortilla with lowfat cheese, plus an orange. Or try a bowl of whole-grain cereal with fat-free milk and a banana.

Break Bad Breakfast Habits

There's a saying that's somewhat true: If you are going to overeat, you might as well do it at breakfast. That way, you have all day to burn off the calories. But overeating calories and fat at any meal, including breakfast, can still hamper your fat-fighting efforts. And some breakfast foods are deceiving. They seem healthy yet are loaded with fat or calories. Here is what you need to know to avoid breakfast fat traps.

Watch your toppings. You can ruin plenty of otherwise healthy foods by putting the wrong things on top of them. Oatmeal is a great fat-fighting breakfast, but adding ¼ cup of half-and-half and 2 teaspoons of margarine brings the meal up to 58 percent fat. So leave off the margarine and replace the cream with fat-free milk.

You can save 19 grams of fat by using an ounce of fat-free cream cheese instead of regular cream cheese on your bagel. And you can slash fat by 28 percent by replacing whole milk with fat-free milk on your cereal.

Make sure your muffins are low-fat. When we see the words *oat bran* or *whole grain*, we think, "Healthy." But that's not always the case. Some oat bran muffins, for instance, are loaded with fat, says Grabowski-Nepa. So be sure to check the label.

Use jelly in moderation. You may be fooled into thinking that all-fruit spreads mean "all you can eat." They don't. Fruit spreads are made with real fruit as well as fruit juice, which is just a nice name for sugar. "Your body can't tell the difference between fruit juice and sugar," says Grabowski-Nepa. Sure, all-fruit spreads are slightly more nutritious than jams and jellies, which can be nearly all processed sugar and very little fruit. But they still have a lot of calories.

Be yogurt smart. When picking yogurt as a breakfast food, pick the right kind. Go for either nonfat or 99 percent fat-free yogurt. And look for one that does not list sugar as an ingredient.

Eat out with caution. Eating at a diner can be a fat and calorie nightmare. A typical waffle, for instance, has 550 calories and 21 grams of fat. Just one slice of French toast has 150 calories and 7 grams of fat. And a single pancake without butter and syrup has 165 calories and 5 grams of fat.

So what can you order? Ask for an egg-white omelet loaded with mushrooms, onions, tomatoes, spinach, or other vegetables. Forgo the cheese and ham. And get some whole-grain toast on the side, says Grabowski-Nepa.

Your Guide to
Sensible Snacking

If you're trying to lose weight, you should snack for precisely the same reason that your mother told you not to when you were a kid: It'll ruin your appetite.

Snacks keep you from overeating at mealtime. That's a good thing. Any time you overeat, your body turns into a fat-storing machine. Snacking also supplies your body with the fuel it needs to keep calories on a steady burn. Without a small snack break every few hours, your stomach gets empty, signaling your metabolism to burn calories more slowly.

But snacking can be risky business. You can't lose weight eating Hershey bars, Twinkies, and Reese's Pieces. The trick to snacking the fat-fighter's way lies in picking the right snack foods. Eating healthy snacks throughout the day that are full of nutrients and fiber and low in fat and calories can help you lose weight because you won't be hungry. You will be able to resist temptation.

Redefining *Snack*

"There's a connotation that snacks must be bad," says Diane Grabowski-Nepa, R.D., nutrition educator at the Pritikin Longevity Center in Malibu, California. "I think we feel that way because of the foods we typically snacked on in the past—usually something sweet or salty. But snacks can be so healthy. You can eat fruit. You can have soup. You can do leftovers. You can have a baked potato. Snacking in itself is healthy. It just depends on what you eat when you snack."

Usually it's taste, not health or weight loss, that controls which snacks we tend to reach for, says Audrey Cross, Ph.D., associate clinical professor of public health at the Columbia University Institute of Human Nutrition in New York City.

How we view taste is a product of upbringing. Most of us reach for snacks that we identify as comfort foods. "We might be bored or feel angry or depressed. Or we might feel we deserve a reward," says Marcia Levin Pelchat, Ph.D., a food-cravings expert at the Monell Chemical Senses Center in Philadelphia. "Then we turn to certain foods that, in our experience, make us feel better." Usually, this means fatty snacks like potato chips and ice cream.

"Fortunately, you can find many snack items like cookies, cakes, and ice cream in low-fat, low-sugar, low-sodium versions," says Dr. Cross. "By choosing these in moderation, our snack urge can be quelled without disastrous nutritional consequences."

Refine Your Tastes

Many people learn to retrain their tastebuds and thus lose interest in fatty, sugary snacks, Dr. Cross says. Does that mean that we can learn to appreciate the color and crunch of a green pepper as much as the gooey richness of a Snickers bar?

"Yes, but for most of us it's not easy," says Dr. Cross. "It takes time. You may fall off the wagon occasionally, but you can do it." Here's how to get started.

Think nutrition. In planning your daily nutrition goals, factor in snacks. "Think of snacks as food eaten between meals instead of as treats or rewards," says Barbara Whedon, R.D., a nutrition counselor at Thomas Jefferson University Hospital in Philadelphia. "Make your snack an extension of your meal. If you plan to have soup, salad, and fruit for lunch, for example, don't eat the fruit. Save it for your snack. The same with your dessert or bread at dinner or your breakfast juice or muffin."

Don't try to be perfect. Denying yourself rarely works, says Margo Denke, M.D., associate professor of internal medicine at the Center for Human Nutrition at the University of Texas Southwestern Medical Center in Dallas. One thing that does, she says, is cutting back on how much you eat when you do snack. Also, don't assume that every single snack you eat has to be nutritious. "Some can be just for fun. It's the overall diet that counts in terms of nutrition," says Dr. Denke.

Plan for temptation. Take your own snacks to work so that when everyone else is selecting an item from the snack cart, you have dried fruit in your desk or nonfat yogurt in your office pantry, says Dr. Cross. "That way, you get something to eat too."

Look for healthier substitutes. If you crave a salty snack, for example, and you're used to appeasing that desire with a bag of potato chips, look for low-fat brands, says Alice K. Lindeman, R.D., Ph.D., associate professor at Indiana University in Bloomington. Just be

"Fat-Free" Pitfalls

When you see "no-fat" in huge letters on a food package, your brain often registers "no-calorie." Unfortunately, those no-fat goodies can be just as high in calories as the regular kinds. For example, when the manufacturers take the fat from a chocolate cookie, they often substitute a whole lot of sugar, making up most if not all of the calories that went away with the fat.

Extra sugar is what makes fat-free cookies taste so good. Since the tendency with fat-free snacks is to eat as much as you want, it's easy to take in a large number of calories. The fat-free claim even makes some people think that eating fat-free snacks will help them lose weight. The problem is that eating more calories than you burn, no matter if those calories come from high-fat or nonfat foods, makes you gain weight and body fat, according to Barbara Whedon, R.D., nutrition counselor at Thomas Jefferson University Hospital in Philadelphia.

The best way to deal with nonfat snacks is to read the fine print. Take a look at the nutrition label, especially the size of the portions and the calorie content of each. No-fat is no lie, but if you do a little extra detective work, you'll be able to make a much more informed decision about how much you really want to eat. Just remember that there can be too much of a good thing when it comes to no-fat noshing, especially if you have a sweet tooth.

careful not to eat more than you used to. An even better choice would be pretzels. "The big Dutch pretzels take a while to eat and can satisfy that desire for salt and crunch," she says.

Beware the Fat Trap

The fact that you eat low-fat snacks doesn't give you license to eat freely of other foods. When Barbara Rolls, Ph.D., professor of nutrition at Pennsylvania State University in University Park, and her colleagues analyzed the impact of such snacks on eating behaviors, they found that those who ate low-fat snacks tended to eat more at lunch than people who ate higher-fat snacks.

"We concluded that thinking a food is low-fat can be a trap because we may believe it gives us license to overindulge in other areas," says Dr. Rolls.

A little math reveals why low-fat snacks can be a trap. Thirteen reduced-fat mini chocolate-chip cookies may add up to only 130 calories. But if you eat the whole 7½-ounce box, you'll take in an amazing 910 calories. It's awfully easy to do that while watching a favorite television show. As another example, you can have 22 low-fat tortilla chips for 110 calories, which sounds great, but the entire 7-ounce package would cost you 770 calories.

"Those grams of fat add up quickly, and so do the calories," Whedon explains. "I tell my clients that eating 40 to 60 grams of fat a day is reasonable. Dropping much below that greatly restricts your food choices and is difficult to maintain. You must make a decision about how many grams of fat you will devote to snacks."

Craving Control

To satisfy your tastebuds, intellectualize your choices, says Whedon. "Often, we grab what's nearby. We feel hungry, so we hurriedly select something from the vending machine or have one of the cookies served at a meeting, with no thought about what we feel a need for," she says.

Think texture. What we often crave is a mouth feel more than a taste, according to Whedon. Snacks can be chewy, crunchy, smooth, creamy, cold, sweet, or salty. Often, we want a combination. "If you crave something creamy and sweet, for example, yogurt might be perfect," says Whedon. "If you desire cold and crunchy, try slices of green pepper. An ice pop will take care of cold and sweet, while Gummi Bears are chewy and sweet."

Plan ahead. "Understand that snacking can be a spontaneous behavior, and be prepared," says Dr. Lindeman. "Keep some items like rice cakes, dried fruit, or cereal mix in a desk drawer, or find a vending machine with healthy selections."

Practice damage control. Don't fall for the notion that if one tastes good, two taste better. Filling a small bowl with potato chips instead of diving into a full bag helps willpower do its work.

Avoid triggers. Boredom can lead to unnecessary snacking. Nutrition experts advise keeping busy when you feel like having a snack. Food commercials and being around people who are eating can also trigger the urge to indulge. Finally, bypass the supermarket aisles loaded with finger foods and the checkout lanes stocked with candy bars, suggests Dr. Cross.

Take slipups in stride. If you do overindulge, forgive yourself, forget about it, and get back on course.

Treat yourself every once in a while. "If you're counting calories, save enough of them to give yourself an occasional treat," says Whedon. "That way, you won't feel deprived, and that will vastly increase your chances of success."

Control your servings. It's easy to overeat on snacks, so choose foods that come in single-serving portions, such as yogurt in 8-ounce cups and pieces of fruit. For low-fat chips and unsalted pretzels, make your own single servings, using snack-size plastic bags.

Think of snacks as golden opportunities to eat the foods you often avoid. For some of us, that's vegetables and

(continued on page 82)

Super No-Fat Snacks

The secret of successful snacking is to be selective. Instead of snacking mindlessly, think about your choices. Here are 50 indulgences that, when eaten in the portions listed, can keep eating fun without packing on the pounds.

Food	Portion	Calories	Fat (g)
Apple	1 medium	81	0
Applesauce, unsweetened	½ cup	53	0
Apricots, dried	5	83	0
Apricots, fresh	3 medium	51	0
Bagel	½	81	0
Banana	1 medium	100	0
Blueberries	1 cup	82	0
Bread, sourdough	1 slice	70	1
Butterscotch candy	4 pieces	88	1
Cantaloupe, cubed	½ cup	57	0
Carrot	1 medium	31	0
Celery	1 stalk	6	0
Cereal, frosted, shredded wheat	4 biscuits	100	0
Cookie, devil's food, low-fat	1	50	0
Cookie, pecan, low-fat	1	70	3
Cottage cheese, low-fat	½ cup	81	1
Crackers, saltines	5	60	1
Crackers, whole-grain, fat-free	5	60	0
Crackers, whole wheat	6	96	3
Cucumber	1 medium	16	0
Dill pickle	1 medium	12	0
Fig bars, fat-free	2	100	0
Fruit juice bar, frozen	1	25	0

Food	Portion	Calories	Fat (g)
Fruit roll candy	1 roll	81	1
Graham cracker	2 squares	60	1
Grapefruit	½ medium	37	0
Grapes	1 cup	58	0
Gummi Bears candy	3 pieces	20	0
Honeydew melon, cubed	1 cup	60	0
Jelly beans	8 large	83	0
LifeSavers candy	1	9	0
Orange	1 medium	65	0
Peach, dried	1	62	0
Peach, fresh	1 medium	37	0
Pepper, green or sweet red	1 large	20	0
Pineapple, cubed	1 cup	77	0
Popcorn, caramel, fat-free	1 cup	110	0
Popcorn, light	1 cup	45	3
Potato chips, fat-free	30	110	0
Pretzel, whole wheat	1 small	51	0
Pretzels	10 thin	70	0
Pudding, chocolate	4 oz	100	0
Raisins, seedless	2 tablespoons	55	0
Rice cake, plain	1	21	0
Strawberries	1 cup	45	0
String cheese, low-fat	1 piece	60	3
Tortilla chips, baked, low-fat, with salsa	10	90	1
Tuna, light, packed in water	2 oz	65	0
Yogurt, nonfat	½ cup	60	0
Yogurt bar, frozen, nonfat	1	45	0

fruits. Some ideas include broccoli florets with low-fat sour cream dip, a baked sweet potato drizzled with fat-free caramel sauce, low-fat tortilla chips with salsa, frozen grapes or bananas, and shredded carrot salad with low-fat mayonnaise and raisins.

Top your popcorn. Air-popped popcorn minus the butter can seem bland. But with a little creativity, it can be a taste treat. Try sprinkling on a little grated cheese or hot spices, like pepper or chili powder. You can even toss in some cinnamon or a handful of raisins.

Guilt-Free, Fun-to-Eat Snacks

Tired of pretzels? Bored with low-fat cookies? Can't look at another carrot? Don't revert to cupcakes just yet. Here are some other tempting snack choices that won't pack fat on your thighs.

• Keep sliced turkey breast in the fridge for sandwiches. Line a pita pocket with lettuce and tuck in the turkey.

• Layer nonfat frozen yogurt with chopped fruit and roasted chestnuts in a sundae dish. Try vanilla yogurt with chopped bananas, or strawberry yogurt with sliced strawberries.

• Toss leftover fresh pasta with a smidgen of olive oil to keep it from clumping, then store it in a sealed plastic bag in the fridge. You can use it to make instant pasta salad by tossing 1 tablespoon of nonfat dressing with 1 cup of pasta. Toss in some leftover vegetables too.

• Make ice cream sandwiches by spreading slightly softened nonfat frozen yogurt between two low-fat oatmeal cookies or graham crackers. Store them, tightly wrapped, in the freezer.

• Peel and section a variety of citrus fruits. For a quick treat, mix grapefruit sections with oranges and tangerines.

• For delicious potato-skin snacks, bake extra potatoes and stash them in the fridge. When you're ready, halve the potatoes and scoop out the insides with a spoon, leaving about ¼ inch of flesh. Sprinkle the skins with shredded reduced-fat Cheddar cheese and minced chives. Broil about 5½ inches from the heat until the potatoes are warmed through and the cheese has melted, about 4 minutes.

• Heat a frozen waffle according to package directions. Top it with maple yogurt, made by folding together equal parts of maple syrup and plain nonfat yogurt. Add sliced bananas or apples.

• For an easy and delicious dip, combine ½ cup of nonfat ricotta and ½ cup of nonfat yogurt. Stir in 1 to 2 teaspoons of your favorite herbs, such as basil, dill, and tarragon. Enjoy with slices of fresh vegetables or reduced-fat whole wheat crackers.

• Nibble on strips of low-fat cheese and strips of sweet red, yellow, and green peppers or chunks of carrots.

• Keep chunks of mangoes and nectarines, plus some seedless grapes and pitted cherries, in plastic bags in the freezer. They're quick refreshers, and they're as good as ice pops.

• Choose some raw vegetables and keep them in bite-size pieces in the fridge. Eat them either with or without a low-fat dip. Cherry tomatoes, sugar snap peas, whole white mushrooms, Jerusalem artichokes, cut-up fennel bulb, Chinese cabbage ribs, sliced celeriac, sliced daikons, and some jicama chunks can perk up your palate.

Leaner Lunches

Besides packing some extra padding on your thighs, a lunch that's high in fat can make you groggy in the afternoon, when you should be mentally alert. So lunch is the perfect meal to eat lean.

In addition to being low in fat, the ideal lunch, whether you are packing it yourself or eating out, should be balanced, says Kathy Dimoff, R.D., former coordinator of the SlimDown Program at St. Elizabeth Health Center in Youngstown, Ohio. That means one fruit, one vegetable, two breads, and a small meat or dairy serving. What's that in real food terms? An apple and a sandwich made with two slices of whole wheat bread, one or two slices of turkey, and some lettuce, tomatoes, sprouts, or even sliced green peppers.

This means that the bulk of your meal will consist of grains, fruits, and vegetables, the hallmark of healthy eating. But there are plenty of ways to get this nutritional balance into your lunch without resorting to a turkey sandwich every day.

Brown-Bag Basics

Packing lunch in these days of hectic living takes time, but would you do it if it earned you $1,000? When Dimoff asked women at her diet center if they would pack their lunches if they were paid $1,000 a day, everyone raised their hand.

"It proves that finding time for packing lunch is just a matter of priority," she says. So put it at the top of your to-do list, with the help of the following advice.

Mondays are for stocking. Put together your lunch staples on Monday mornings. That means taking foods like bananas, canned soup, pretzels, apples, small cans of applesauce, and dry cereal to work and storing them for the week to come.

Build a good sandwich. Just one sandwich can contain everything you want to eat for lunch: bread, vegetables, and protein, points out Dimoff. Here's her advice for mastering sandwich making.

• Choose whole-grain bread or pitas. Because they have more fiber, whole-grain breads fill you up faster than their white counterparts.

• Skip the usual deli meats and choose lean cuts of chicken, turkey, or roast beef. Your serving of meat should weigh no more than 3 ounces.

• Go wild with vegetables. Pile on any combination of sprouts, sliced cucumbers, green pepper rings, shredded carrots, onions, sliced mushrooms, romaine lettuce, and shredded cabbage. The vegetables add moisture to your sandwich, eliminating the need for mayonnaise.

Have a pita party. For something a little more festive, make some bean dip or buy ready-made hummus and pack it in a plastic container. For dipping, slice a pita and wrap it separately.

Bring on the soup. A vegetable-based soup can also be a perfect lunch if you round it out with some bread or fat-free crackers and fruit. Plus, it has a bonus: You'll eat less. A study at the obesity research center at St. Luke's–Roosevelt Hospital in New York City showed that when people have soup for lunch, they eat less at that meal and feel more satisfied.

Because soup is hot, you eat it more slowly, explains Judith S. Stern, R.D., Sc.D., professor of nutrition and internal medicine at the University of California at Davis. So your brain has the time to tell your stomach, "I'm full." Home-made soup is ideal, but canned soup is fine provided you check the label to make sure the fat count is low, she says.

Have dinner for lunch. Here's a real time-saver: Lunch on the leftovers from the previous night's dinner. "If you are making salmon steaks, for instance, prepare an extra one," says Marie Simmons, author of *Fresh and Fast* and monthly food columnist for the magazine *Bon Appétit*. "Salmon is good cold, and you can round it out with a salad of cooked potatoes and cucumber slices drizzled with a little lemon juice and olive oil."

Break tradition. There's no reason you can't have a totally nontraditional brown-bag lunch. How about a single-serving box of your favorite whole-grain cereal topped with nonfat yogurt or fat-free milk, along with some cut-up fruit?

Lunchtime Survival

Brown-bagging may be the best way to go, but let's be realistic: You probably won't make your own lunch every day. Whether you're venturing out to a restaurant or heading to the company cafeteria for lunch, these strategies can help you eat great and lose weight.

Start off with a snack. Before lunching out, have a snack from the low-fat stash in your desk drawer. This will take the edge off your hunger so you won't be dipping bread into olive oil while waiting for your food.

Escape the Salad Bar Fat Trap

Salads are the staple of many dieters, and rightfully so—they can be both healthy and filling. But by adding regular salad dressing and a lot of cheese, eggs, and croutons to a plate of lettuce, you can mire yourself in the salad bar fat trap.

Suppose you typically lunch on a turkey sandwich made of two slices of cracked-wheat bread, two slices of turkey, 2 teaspoons of regular mayonnaise, and a little lettuce and tomato. Throw in a cup of vegetable soup on the side and your lunch contains about 375 calories and 14 grams of fat. That's not bad. If you get out a big salad bowl and pile up some lettuce, cheese, turkey, egg, croutons, crunchy vegetables, and 2 tablespoons of Caesar dressing, you have a lunch with 600 calories and 36 grams of fat. So much for your hopes of dropping a few pounds.

Salad can be a healthy way to go, especially when you add a lot of vegetables. It's just not going to help you lose weight unless you cut back on the high-fat salad bar fixings, according to Neva Cochran, R.D., private nutrition consultant and American Dietetic Association spokesperson in Dallas.

The key to making a leaner lunch is to pay attention to portion size. When you're trying to fight fat, soups, salads, and sandwiches are all satisfactory choices; you just have to avoid serving up anything with fattening frills and on a huge plate. *

Be a leader. When lunching with friends, be assertive and voice your restaurant preference. Have two or three alternatives in mind, places where you know they serve at least one reduced-fat meal.

Get familiar with the menu. Whenever possible, go to restaurants you're familiar with so that before leaving the office you can make up your mind about what you're going to eat. That way, you can order without having to look at a menu that's just begging you to change your mind.

Dine alone. It may be kind of lonely, but you'll eat less. Psychologists theorize that you linger over your food and eat more when you're with company. Researchers at Georgia State University in Atlanta found that when people ate with one companion, their consumption rose by 28 percent. With two companions, they ate 41 percent more, and with six or more companions, they ate 76 percent more food.

Go to a deli. With tons of fattening stuff like corned beef, bologna, cheese, and pepperoni, delis may at first seem like the last places you'd want to eat lunch. But a deli is actually one of your best options, says Toni Ferrang, R.D., owner of Food for Thought Nutrition Consulting in the San Francisco Bay area. You have more choices and more freedom to custom order than at any other type of restaurant. You don't have to order the six-different-kinds-of-meat-and-cheese submarine sandwich slathered with mayo and oil. Instead, you can get a turkey sandwich with tomato, lettuce, and mustard on whole wheat bread.

Do a balancing act. There will be times when you simply won't be able to choose what you eat. At a conference, for instance, the menu may be a predetermined mix of fatty foods. Just eat modest portions, says Dimoff.

Take a taste of temptation. Ah, the smell of those wonderful hot dogs you love so much from the cart on the corner is luring you into temptation. Well, let it once in a while. Sure, the dogs are full of fat, but if you make smart food choices the rest of the day, you'll stay out of fat city. Just round out each of your meals with a piece of fruit or a vegetable, says Ferrang.

Svelte Suppers

Dinner is the meal most likely to destroy a diet.

In reality, the problem is not dinner. Those who splurge during or after dinner usually can trace their true food problem to much earlier in the day. "Their biggest problem is breakfast and lunch because they skip them or eat very little," says Toni Ferrang, R.D., owner of Food for Thought Nutrition Consulting in the San Francisco Bay area. "By the time dinner comes around, they're so hungry they're all over the food."

If you're a night eater and you want to lose weight, you're going to have to turn your eating habits nearly upside-down. Night eating is the worst thing you can do, says Ferrang, because what you overeat at night will very likely follow you to bed. And since your body goes on slow burn while you sleep, those calories will look for a cozy place to rest too—right in your fat cells. So you have to toss some of those extra supper calories toward your breakfast and lunch, spreading your calorie intake more evenly throughout the day, says Ferrang. Here's what she suggests.

The Dinner Knell

Once you start eating more during the day, you'll have solved more than three-quarters of your dinner dilemma, says Ferrang. What's the remaining quarter? Your dining companions.

Putting smaller, low-fat dinners on the table can get dicey when you have a meat-hungry family to feed. It's even trickier when you have picky kids who cringe at the sight of vegetables, whole grains, and just about anything low-fat and nutritious. With some communication, compromise, and even sheer trickery, however, you can stick to your food plan while keeping others happy.

Tell them your intentions. If you are watching what you eat but others keep tempting you with second helpings, explain how you are trying to eat and why. Chances are, once they understand, they'll be more supportive, says Ferrang.

Another tack is to try to strike a compromise, suggests Joyce D. Nash, Ph.D., a clinical psychologist in San Francisco and Palo Alto, California, and author of *The New Maximize Your Body Potential*. Maybe the others can go out for pizza, burgers, or hot dogs once a week, for instance. Or get them to cook meals for themselves a couple of nights a week while you fend for yourself.

Remember, you have the right to eat whatever you want, even if your family doesn't want the same things. You can strike a balance between the meals everyone likes and the meals you need. You don't need to please everyone all the time. Sometimes, it's good to just not worry about what they say.

Fill up on vegetables. You can continue to fix the meat your family loves while at the same time cutting back on fatty foods. Just be sure to cook up a bunch of vegetables and whole grains, says Marsha Hudnall, R.D., director of nutrition programs at Green Mountain at Fox Run, a health and weight-management community for women in

Ludlow, Vermont. If others crave steak, for instance, go ahead and make it. Just make sure it's a lean cut, limit yourself to a 3-ounce portion (that's about the size of your palm), and fill the rest of your plate with broccoli, brown rice, and steamed carrots, she says.

Cook up an optical illusion. A small amount of meat looks like a lot when you cut it into small pieces and mix it with a bunch of stir-fried vegetables, says Hudnall.

Similarly, try fixing a stew with lots of vegetables, a delicious broth, and only a little meat, says Diane Woznicki, R.D., a nutritionist at the University of Pennsylvania in Philadelphia. Or try making a pasta or rice dish and garnishing it with thinly sliced beef or chicken. The same goes for fajitas: Use lots of peppers and onions but only three strips or so of meat. You'll feel like you're getting a treat while you meet your weight-loss requirements.

Pull a disappearing act. Those who hate vegetables can't complain if they don't know what they are eating. Try finely chopping or pureeing vegetables and hiding them in family favorites such as meat loaf and tacos. To make tacos, for instance, Hudnall stretches a small amount of lower-fat ground beef by mixing in tomato paste and finely chopped celery and onions. "The tacos end up having a lot of vegetables, but the kids don't know it," Hudnall says.

Tempt with color. "I often tell people to cook by color and to include a variety of fruits and vegetables that are red, green, yellow, and orange," says Pat Baird, R.D., author of *The Pyramid Cookbook*. And orange doesn't restrict you to oranges. There are cantaloupes, apricots, papayas, mangoes, winter squash, and orange peppers.

Persist for 10 dinners. You know how people talk about having an "acquired taste" for beer, coffee, or caviar? The same thing can happen with vegetables. Once you eat a food about 10 times, you'll learn to like it, says Hudnall.

Beware of Subtle Eating Cues

Here are simple changes you can make in your eating environment to help you eat less without even thinking about it.

Set a dark table. Bright colors such as orange, red, and yellow make you hungry, according to research at Johns Hopkins Medical Institutions in Baltimore. But darker colors such as gray, black, or brown don't. Although your kitchen won't look as warm with a dark tablecloth, dark napkins, or dark walls, they could help your weight-loss efforts.

Eat from small packages. If a food comes in a large package, you will most likely use more of it, according to research from the University of Pennsylvania in Philadelphia. The moral is that the smaller the bottles of cooking oil, packages of sweets, and boxes of food you buy, the less you'll eat during each sitting.

Munch to Mozart, not syndicated sitcoms. Listening to gentle music while you dine forces you to concentrate on

Low-Fat Cooking Secrets

Low-fat food doesn't have to be tasteless and rubbery. You can discover new delights, not grim restrictions, on a low-fat dinner eating plan, says nutrition counselor Michelle Berry, R.D., research nutritionist at the University of Pittsburgh. "If you think about getting variety in flavors, ingredients, and preparation styles, healthy eating can be a delicious, satisfying adventure," she says.

In fact, if you concentrate on making small changes, you can slowly eliminate fat from your favorite dishes. And no one will even notice, says Kathy Dimoff, R.D., former coordinator of the SlimDown Program at St. Elizabeth Health Center in Youngstown, Ohio. Here are ways to cut the fat out of your dinners without sacrificing flavor or satisfaction.

what you are eating, which means you'll eat more slowly and eat less. You'll also be more satisfied because slowing down allows you to taste the food. If you eat while watching television, eating becomes automatic, so you eat more.

Channel surf away the commercials. If you do eat while watching television, be extra careful if a diet commercial pops up. In one study, 86 women dieters drank a milkshake and then watched a sad movie with either no commercials, neutral commercials, or ones featuring successful dieters. The women were supposed to test bowls of peanuts and M&M's during the flick. The women who saw the diet commercials ate nearly twice as much as the other women. Researchers suspect that the thin women in the ads reminded the women who watched that they had gone off their diets, which removed their inhibitions about eating.

Take fat from your favorites. Most cooks use the same 10 or so recipes over and over again. So pull together your regulars, look them over, and find ways to eliminate fat. "You can often make very subtle changes that another person will never notice," says Dimoff. Changes could include substituting extra-lean ground beef or turkey for the higher-fat variety, using lower-fat dairy products, and mixing in more spices and less oil.

Investing in a quality no-stick skillet means that you won't have to add as much oil to sauté food, says Ferrang.

Try broth. Instead of sautéing in oil, try using vegetable or chicken broth, says Ferrang.

Fry without the fat. Generally, frying is the worst way to cook anything. That's because your food is simply sitting in butter or oil, absorbing all that pure liquid fat and delivering it straight to your belly. Two fried favorites, chicken and french fries, can be made without the grease, says Dimoff. To make fries, slice baking potatoes into wedges, sprinkle with ground red pepper, and roast in the oven until brown. You'll save 12 grams of fat per serving. To make chicken, dip skinless breasts in egg whites and roll them in bread crumbs, then bake.

Let it soak. Marinate your fish or meat in soy or teriyaki sauce ahead of time to add flavor. That way, you won't feel tempted to fry it, says Ferrang.

Get the best cut. When it comes to red meat, choose leaner cuts such as loin and round. A top round steak contains 3 grams of fat per 3-ounce serving, while a rib-eye steak contains 10 grams per 3 ounces.

Cut the fat. Always trim visible fat from meat before cooking. It can make a big difference. Three ounces of beef chuck pot roast, for example, has 18 grams of fat. Trimmed, the same cut has 6 grams.

Spray. Use cooking spray instead of oil or butter. You'll save on fat no matter what you're cooking.

Turn the dial first. If you heat the skillet before adding oil, less fat will be absorbed by the food. Warm oil cooks more efficiently, while cold oil tends to soak into meats and vegetables.

Learn pseudo-sautéing. Instead of letting your food swim in a puddle of oil, cook it with its own natural moisture. Begin with the tiniest quantity of oil and add water, not more oil, for moisture as needed.

When you roast meat, use a rack. A rack allows fat to drip off so the meat doesn't steep in it and reabsorb all the bad stuff.

Know your marinades. When grilling chicken, try this oil-free marinade: Combine 3 cups of apple juice and two cloves of garlic, minced, with 1 cup of reduced-sodium soy sauce. Experiment with making other marinades without fat. Try flavored vinegars, fruit juices, and a variety of spices and herbs.

Have some spicy low-fat Buffalo wings. Instead of using chicken wings, use skinless chicken breast tenders to make "Buffalo wings." Marinate them overnight in the refrigerator in a mixture of hot-pepper sauce, olive oil, lots of garlic powder, and red wine vinegar. (Experiment with the amounts to suit your taste.) Then roast the chicken wings at 400°F for 15 minutes.

Be a low-fat loafer. Make a better meat loaf using a mixture of one-third cooked brown rice or oatmeal, one-third ground turkey (breast meat only), and one-third extra-lean beef. Splash on Worcestershire sauce, barbecue sauce, or ketchup. You won't miss the missing fat.

Make chicken à l'orange. If you have a can of frozen orange juice concentrate, you have a great way to add flavor to stir-fried chicken or beef and vegetables without adding fat. Just a few spoonfuls will do.

Perk up your corn. Stir salsa into frozen corn while you heat it through; the spice eliminates the need for butter. When you're boiling corn on the cob, add some ground red pepper to the water for butter-free Cajun corn.

Slim down your pasta sauce. If you're making your own spaghetti sauce, look for the seasoned, stewed varieties of canned tomatoes. They tend to be lower in oil than those labeled pasta-ready. You can also use frozen veggie burger crumbles instead of ground beef.

If it's Friday, this must be pizza. Pizza is one of those foods that many people crave almost as much as meat, so you probably won't hear any complaints about this meal. Try homemade pizza that boasts a low-fat crust topped with low-fat cheese and steamed vegetables. It can go a long way toward meeting your remaining nutritional requirements for the day, says Cheryl Rock, Ph.D., associate professor of nutrition in the department of family and preventive medicine at the University of California, San Diego, School of Medicine.

Or try a fruit pizza. Start with a low-fat whole wheat pastry crust. Mix fat-free cream cheese with low-fat or nonfat ricotta and spread it over the baked crust. Add ki-

---

Q & A

Why Do Men Love Meat-and-Potato Meals?

Many men say they crave protein. They say that a vegetarian meal just can't satisfy their hunger like a good, juicy steak and a nice, buttery baked potato can. But most men who think a meal isn't a meal without meat and potatoes think so because their fathers were also meat-and-potatoes men. If a woman comes from a household where dinner was dictated by her father's appetite, she could conceivably be a meat-and-potato lover too.

It's all about foods that we considered familiar in the past—comfort foods. To deal with those who turn up their noses at anything that doesn't qualify, start by choosing alternatives to meat that they're likely to respond to. Serving tofu 7 days a week won't do it, but there's room for compromise—say, a supper of pasta with vegetables or fish, or poultry with rice.

Enlist meat eaters in the process of buying and preparing food, cut down on meaty meals gradually, and maybe even promise one "real" meal a week. The key, however, is to convince them that meat-free meals *are* real meals.

Expert consulted: Jeanne Goldberg, R.D., Ph.D., associate professor and director, graduate program in nutrition communication, School of Nutrition Science and Policy, Tufts University, Boston

wifruit or other fruits—peaches, berries, and so forth—as if they were pepperoni. Heat some marmalade in the microwave and brush it on top with a pastry brush, then enjoy.

Portion Control

Even if you successfully jump on the low-fat dinner wagon, you still have one more obstacle to tackle: portion size. Here are some strategies.

Sigh. Really. Take a deep breath before actually picking up your fork for the first bite. It will help you to relax, eat more slowly, and stop before you stuff yourself.

Cover your plate. Many people overeat at dinner because they skimp on their initial servings. They put only a little of this and a tiny bit of that on their plates. Then they eat that tiny bit. "They feel like that was nothing, so they go back for more," says Hudnall. But serving number two is larger. And serving number three is still larger. Eventually, they end up stuffed but still unsatisfied.

Instead, fill up your plate the first time, covering the majority with lower-calorie vegetables and grains. The simple act of covering the dish can make you mentally satisfied, Hudnall says. And you won't be tempted by seconds.

Stay seated. Try this dinner exercise: Set your kitchen timer for 20 minutes. Then don't allow yourself to get up from the table until it goes off, says Dimoff. This exercise will make you realize how quickly you eat, she says. It takes about 20 minutes for your brain to realize that you have swallowed food. So if you eat more slowly, you're less likely to accidentally stuff yourself.

Focus on food. Focusing on tasting and smelling what you eat will help you to eat more slowly, which will help you to eat less. Remember to sit down, turn off the television, and put your fork down between bites, says Ferrang.

Taking Your Diet Out to Eat

Restaurants are famous for serving portions that only King Kong could finish. But that doesn't mean you can't find sensible meals outside of your own kitchen. If you master four simple fat-fighting strategies, you should be able to eat out whenever you want, enjoy your food, and not gain a pound, says Elizabeth Brown, R.D., nutritionist and weight-control specialist at the Lehigh Valley Hospital Center for Health Promotion and Disease Prevention in Allentown, Pennsylvania. The best strategies for eating out, feeling satisfied, and fighting fat are thinking, choosing, ordering, and eating, in that order.

Dining-Out Art #1: Think Ahead

Much of the secret to eating out lies in what you do before you set foot out of your house. You want to be in control when you arrive at the restaurant. That means already knowing that you are going to order a healthy, low-fat meal. Here's how to plan.

Wear something nice but form-fitting. A precision-fitted waistband reminds you to practice portion control. It sounds crazy, but it works, says Susan Olson, Ph.D., a clinical psychologist and weight-management consultant in Seattle and author of *Keeping It Off: Winning at Weight Loss.* "Your focus shifts from the sensations of the taste, smell, and sight of the food to your body and how you want to look," she says.

Ruin your appetite. Yes, it's perfectly okay—in fact, it's smart—to have a low-cal snack or beverage at home before leaving for the restaurant. The snack tames your hunger pangs so you don't gorge later on. Good choices include a few crackers with low-fat cheese or a small green salad with a bit of fat-free dressing. "This technique works on the same principle as not going to the grocery store hungry," says Dr. Olson. "If you eat a little before you leave the house, you'll be able to make rational choices in the restaurant instead of just eating out of hunger."

Visualize yourself eating wisely. Mentally rehearse what you will order. "What you put in your mind is what your brain will follow," says Dr. Olson.

Work off the calories. If you know there's a bigger-than-usual meal in your future, exercise will help burn those extra calories. And there's a bonus: If you take your brisk stroll or quick run before dining out, you'll remember the effort that went into the workout and you'll be less likely to overdo it at mealtime.

Jot down tomorrow's menu today. Think of a restaurant meal as one of 21 healthy meals you expect to eat this week. To help you see this meal in perspective, write down what you plan to eat tomorrow and realize that you're not going to be happy if you have to cut back on tomorrow's food because of today's splurge.

Think about the trip home. How are you going to feel later as you're dabbing your lips with your napkin and getting up from the table? Satisfied or fat? You should feel pleasantly satisfied, never unpleasantly stuffed.

Dining-Out Art #2: Make the Right Choices

Even though restaurants feature large portions and numerous fatty dishes, owners have become increasingly sensitive and responsive to the public's growing demand for low-fat, low-calorie meals. Many have adjusted their menus accordingly. That's why you see more and more restaurants—especially those that cater to businesspeople, who dine out much more than most of us—offering special "heart-smart" and weight-conscious dishes prepared with less saturated fat, less sugar, and more fresh fruits and vegetables.

You'll want to make careful choices about where you'll eat and what you'll order. Here are some factors to take into consideration.

Pick the right kind. It's wise to steer clear of old-fashioned American or home-style restaurants as well as classic French establishments, which have pretty rich dishes, and Continental restaurants, which usually feature heavy sauces and big portions of starches and meats, says Aliza Green, a Philadelphia restaurant consultant and former chef. Her recommendation is ethnic eateries, including Thai, Chinese, Italian, Mediterranean, Greek, Turkish, North African, and the like. "In most ethnic places, you can get a lot more vegetables and grains and lighter sauces, and the more authentic the restaurant, the better." Of course, she warns, "you still have to be careful. In some Italian restaurants, for example, the most popular dish is fettuccine Alfredo, which is loaded with cream and butter."

Get the lower-fat entrées. From fast food to Chinese, just about every type of restaurant has at least one edible lower-fat dish. According to nutritionists, here are some safe picks.

- Mexican: Chicken fajitas and chicken burritos, but skip the guacamole and sour cream

- Fast food: Salad with low-fat dressing, the grilled-chicken sandwich, or the smallest burger without mayonnaise and special sauce
- Deli: A turkey breast or lean roast beef sandwich with mustard
- Italian: Spaghetti with red or white clam sauce
- Chinese: Szechuan shrimp, stir-fried vegetables, shrimp in garlic sauce, or chicken chow mein, all prepared with just a little oil
- Pizzeria: Pizza with vegetable toppings instead of pepperoni, sausage, or extra cheese; and the hand-tossed crust instead of the deep-dish version

Know the language. There are particular key words and phrases on a restaurant menu that generally spell trouble for dieters. Here are some menu words to stay away from: buttery, buttered, butter sauce, sautéed, fried, pan-fried, breaded, glazed, crispy, creamy, creamed, in cream sauce, in its own gravy, au gratin, Parmesan, in cheese sauce, escalloped, au lait, à la mode, au fromage, stewed, basted, prime, hash, pot pie, Hollandaise, deep-fried, dipped in batter, batter-fried, tempura, bisque, Alfredo (butter-and-cheese sauce), carbonara (butter-and-cheese sauce plus bacon), casserole (could contain undetermined, and often rich, sauces or other fatty ingredients), stuffed with cheese or meat, large, extra-large, jumbo, piled-high or stacked, and—last but not least—all you can eat.

Does it sound like there's nothing left? Here's a list of words to eat by: pickled, tomato sauce, cocktail sauce, steamed, poached, in broth, in its own juice, garden fresh, roasted, stir-fried, broiled, charbroiled, grilled, roasted, braised or baked, Florentine (spinach), primavera (with vegetables; this is fine if it's not in cream sauce), marinara (tomato sauce), and stuffed with vegetables or herbs.

Try many restaurants. While one deli may make a corned beef sandwich with plenty of whole-grain bread, lots of relish and sauerkraut, and corned beef with excess fat trimmed off, the next might make one with fatty corned beef, high-calorie Thousand Island dressing, and mounds of cheese. Rather than avoid all of one type of restaurant, shop around. Do a little menu investigating. You can check out all of the Mexican places, for example, and then decide on the healthiest. Just avoid the obvious fry pits where the restaurant counter is a window on the side of a trailer and the cashier wears a stained paper hat.

Appetize lightly. Generally, you want to stay away from fried vegetables and cheese. Instead, opt for clear broth soups, fresh vegetables, or shrimp cocktail. Vegetable and bean soups are often good choices because they are filling. Just avoid any soup with a name beginning with "cream of," says Brown.

Know your salads. Don't let the word *salad* on the menu lull you into thinking that it's automatically a wise choice, says Green. Caesar salad, for example, is the most popular salad in American restaurants. "But it's one of the worst things you can order," she says. "Chefs use mayonnaise and cheese in the dressing, and plenty of it. And the croutons are fried in oil." Similarly, salad bars may look like safe havens for dieters, but watch out. Ladling on those creamy, high-fat dressings, sprinkling on handfuls of croutons or bacon bits, and gobbling down mayonnaise-packed potato and macaroni salads can turn your light meal into a caloric nightmare.

Watch the sidelines. Sometimes, the fattiest part of a restaurant meal isn't the main course or dessert; it's the side dish. Be sure to order vegetables that are steamed, not cooked with butter or cream sauce. And watch what you put on your vegetables once they arrive at the table. You're better off using sour cream rather than butter on

Your Restaurant Survival Guide

Here are 10 ways to enhance your dining experience while lowering the numbers you see on the scale.

1. Before you leave for the restaurant, drink a glass of water or club soda and have a celery stalk or a carrot to take the edge off your hunger.
2. When your dining companions suggest French food (or pizza or ribs), say, "Hmmm, how about seafood (or vegetarian or Thai food) instead?"
3. Instead of attacking the bread basket when you sit down, drink the water poured for you. Then get your companions' okay to ask the waiter to remove the bread and butter.
4. Order tomato juice or mineral water instead of wine.
5. Ignore what everyone else is ordering and just focus on your own meal. In fact, don't even open the menu—you know what you can eat.
6. If you're unsure about how a dish is prepared, ask the server about it and possibly ask to have it changed, say, from fried to baked, or with the sauce on the side.
7. Instead of eating and eating and eating, eat and talk and eat and talk.
8. Leave about half of your meat or fish and ask to have it wrapped so you can take it home.
9. Order some sorbet for dessert and have just a forkful of a companion's cheesecake.
10. Walk home (or take a brisk walk once you get there).

your baked potato, for instance, because a tablespoon of butter has more than four times more fat than a table-spoon of sour cream. Other options include a little low-fat ranch dressing or some grated Parmesan cheese.

Have dessert. You don't have to say no automatically when the dessert cart is wheeled over, says Hope S. War-shaw, R.D., author of *The Restaurant Companion: A Guide to Healthier Eating Out.* "Depending on the restaurant, you can opt for various sweets that are kind to your waistline. Try sorbet. Or lemon ice, which is offered in some Italian restau-rants." Other options, says Warshaw, are fresh raspberries or strawberries with a bit of liqueur. "Also, some family-style restaurants offer low-fat frozen yogurt," she adds.

Bypass the buffet table. Try to steer clear of those one-price, all-you-can-eat joints. If at some point you get stuck at one of these places, don't begin filling your plate until you first look over all the selections. Then choose the lower-fat items. Be sure to start your meal with a broth soup to fill up. Limit yourself to one trip to the buffet, says Brown.

Cut loose occasionally. As a general rule, dining out doesn't mean leaving your diet at home. However—and this is not a contradictory statement—even those who are trying to lose weight are entitled to have exactly what they want in a restaurant from time to time. If you're going out to celebrate your 25th anniversary or your son's college graduation, have that piece of chocolate cake or a glass of champagne. As long as you're mindful of your weight-loss program and return to it immediately, you can have a "sinful" restaurant meal occasionally.

Dining-Out Art #3: Customize Your Order

To fight fat, you'll want to give the server detailed in-structions on how you want to have your food prepared and served. At first, you may feel awkward, but as you get used to being specific about the food you order, it will feel more like second nature. Here are some special considerations to help you have a fat-conscious meal.

Take it on the side. Never let the server ladle dressings, sauces, or gravy onto your food. "Salad dressing is the largest source of fat in many people's diets," says Jayne Hurley, R.D., senior nutritionist with the Center for Science in the Public Interest in Washington, D.C. If a salad comes with avocado, grated cheese, bacon bits, and blue cheese dressing, for instance, you can ask the server to hold the cheese and serve the dressing on the side. Then add just a little bit of dressing for taste. Also, ask for some vinegar on the side to water down the dressing.

If you don't see it, ask for it. "Don't be afraid to make special requests," says Carole Livingston, a frequent restaurant goer and the author of *I'll Never Be Fat Again*. Nine out of 10 restaurant owners surveyed by the National Restaurant Association said that if customers requested it, they would happily serve dishes with sauce or dressing on the side and cook with vegetable oil or margarine instead of highly saturated butter, lard, or shortening. And 8 out of 10 of these eager-to-please restaurateurs added that they would gladly bake or broil chicken or fish rather than fry it.

"If you don't see a simple pasta dish on the menu, for example, but you do see that the restaurant serves other dishes that contain pasta or tomatoes or vegetables, ask for pasta prepared with vegetables in a tomato-based sauce," says Livingston. "Ask the chef to put things together. Often, the better the restaurant, the easier it is to make alternate choices."

Ban the butter. Ask your dining companions if it's okay to move the complimentary bread and butter to their side of the table. Better yet, have the server remove them altogether.

Be wise about size. Don't think that just because you paid for the food, you have to finish every morsel. Ask for a doggie bag and take the rest of the food home for another meal. In fact, have the server put half of your meal in a take-home container before the food is actually served. That way, you won't be tempted to eat the whole thing.

Order first. By doing so, you'll be less tempted to have some of the other, more fattening dishes that your companions may choose.

Ask questions about the menu. To avoid confusion, some people are better off not looking at the menu. If you've been watching what you eat for any length of time, you already have a pretty good idea of what you can have and what you can't. Ask for specifics about the specials; even if they don't have exactly what you want, at the vast majority of restaurants you can still get baked or broiled poultry or fish, a simple pasta dish, steamed vegetables, and fruit for dessert. Remember, the menu is there to tempt you, but you're there to make choices.

Milk it. Ask the server to bring you fat-free milk for your coffee. Unless you ask, you can expect to be served cream or half-and-half.

Make a side dish your entrée. You don't have to order an entrée. Instead, try appetizers or side dishes as a main course.

Dining-Out Art #4: Eat with Pleasure

Once your food arrives on the plate, you can still take some steps to ensure that you won't take fat home on your thighs. Here's how to dine like a fat fighter.

Look around. Remember to take in the atmosphere. Is there a fireplace? Do you like the artwork on the walls? What kind of flowers are on the table? How is your conversation going? All these things can enhance your dining pleasure as well as help you eat more slowly. The result is that you'll eat less.

Breathe deeply. Often when we go out to eat, we focus our attention on how long it's taking the server to bring us our meals. Then, when our food finally comes, we devour it without tasting it. This time, when the server puts your food on the table, don't pick up your fork right away. Instead, pause and enjoy the appearance and aroma of the food for a few seconds, then remind yourself to relax and eat slowly.

Satisfy your thirst. Drink plenty of water throughout the meal—you'll eat less. Order a bottle of mineral water for the table or ask the server to bring a pitcher of tap water.

Go native. In a Chinese or Thai restaurant, use the chopsticks (especially if you don't use them well). It will slow you down, and you'll get full before you can eat the whole meal.

Lose the race. Have an unspoken competition with your dining partners to be the last person to finish eating. Men and women with weight problems tend to eat fast and are usually the first ones in any given group to be finished.

Focus on chatting, not chewing. Talking more and eating less is the secret to enjoying your meal without overindulging, says Dr. Olson.

Dessert Selections You Can Live With

What foods are on your "forbidden" list? How about cheesecake, chocolate, pudding, ice cream, cupcakes, and cookies? Indeed, today's forbidden list usually consists of desserts. And it sets us up for trouble, says Susan Olson, Ph.D., a clinical psychologist and weight-management consultant in Seattle and coauthor of *Keeping It Off: Winning at Weight Loss.*

"The minute you say you can't have something, it becomes especially appealing," says Dr. Olson. "Then, if you do eat it, you'll probably binge, thinking that you should get it while you can. On the other hand, once you know you can have that food, you won't want it as often."

So instead of banning particular foods from your diet, isolate your true passion foods. Then be sure to work those passions into your diet and cut back on other foods that you won't miss, says Toni Ferrang, R.D., owner of Food for Thought Nutrition Consulting in the San Francisco Bay area. If chocolate is your passion, for instance, pick a satisfying portion—say, two or three Godivas—and be sure to have it on selected days, says Dr. Olson.

Sampling what you like most helps you avoid binge eating. But eating small amounts of dessert on a regular basis can also cut down on unnecessary snacking, says Dr. Olson. When you eat something sweet after a meal, you provide your brain with the signal it needs to know that the meal is over. Without something sweet, you may not feel satisfied. And you'll be searching through the kitchen all night, looking for something to munch on.

Halving Your Cake and Eating It Too

When you're working desserts into your fat-fighting plan, you need to pay attention to the portion size and fat content. Here's how.

Follow the law of fours. Ask yourself, "Do I need dessert every day? Do I physically crave it that often?" The answer is probably no, says Denise T. Garner, R.D., instructor of nutrition at York College in Pennsylvania. So instead of having dessert every day, aim to have it four times a week, she says. Then make your dessert days coincide with your exercise days. That way, you won't feel guilty about indulging.

Don't eat fat you don't need. Just as you don't want something sweet every day of the week, you probably don't physically crave the sweetest, fattiest dessert you can think of as often as four times a week, says Garner. So on the dessert days when your tongue isn't telling you to eat cheesecake, chocolate chip cookies, or fudge, go for lower-fat sweets such as fig bars, fruit, fat-free frozen yogurt, sherbet, angel food cake, or gingersnaps, she says. Try making a fresh fruit sundae with low-fat ice milk or frozen yogurt and berries, for instance.

Satisfy your sweet tooth with fruit. Few things taste as refreshing as fresh, seasonal fruit. You can puree fresh fruits like strawberries, then pour the mixture into ice cube trays and freeze it. Or you can make a fruit shake by mixing sliced bananas, fat-free milk, cinnamon, and vanilla in a blender. To make it easy to quickly whip up fruit shakes, keep peeled, sliced fruit in plastic bags in your freezer. When you crave a shake, you can just puree the fruit in a food processor until smooth.

Bake a less fattening cake. One trick to creating wonderful, light desserts without sacrificing taste is to take a favorite recipe and make a few clever substitutions for high-fat and high-sugar ingredients. Fruit juice, for example, can add considerably more flavor than plain old white sugar. Cocoa powder is a fill-in for full-fat chocolate. And marshmallow cream, used instead of butter or margarine, makes a rich, creamy, low-fat frosting. Pureed prunes moisten any chocolate recipe so you don't need as much butter or shortening. (If a recipe calls for 1 cup of butter, use ⅔ cup of prune puree and ⅓ cup of butter. If you don't want to puree the prunes yourself, you can buy prune butter or baby-food prunes.) And if your recipe includes nuts, toast them first at 350°F to intensify their flavor, and then use fewer than the recipe calls for. Here's a list of quick and easy substitutions.

- 1 cup of evaporated fat-free milk instead of 1 cup of heavy cream
- 1 cup of fat-free milk instead of 1 cup of whole milk
- ¼ cup of fat-free egg substitute instead of one medium whole egg
- 3 tablespoons of cocoa powder dissolved in 2 tablespoons of water and mixed with 1 tablespoon of prune puree instead of 1 ounce of baking chocolate
- ½ cup of fruit puree plus ½ cup butter instead of 1 cup of butter (for baking)

- ½ cup of applesauce, or ¼ cup of applesauce and ¼ cup of buttermilk, instead of ½ cup of oil (for baking)
- 1 cup of plain nonfat yogurt instead of 1 cup of sour cream
- ½ cup of marshmallow cream instead of ½ cup of butter (for frosting)
- ½ to ¾ cup of chocolate chips instead of 1 cup of chocolate chips
- 1 teaspoon of coconut flavoring instead of 1 cup of shredded coconut

Do three bites. On days when you crave the likes of Death by Chocolate, take your chosen dessert—yes, any dessert—and have three normal-size bites. When you take the first bite, don't swallow right away. Hold it in your mouth. Let it slowly melt on your tongue. Enjoy it. Really taste it. Then take two more bites exactly the same way. Wrap up whatever is left and save it for the next day. "I always tell people to pick whatever they want because it satisfies them more. Then limit the portion," says Diane Wilke, R.D., a nutrition consultant in Columbus, Ohio.

Fine-tune your portion vision. Prepackaged desserts tell you how many servings make up a cake or pie. When most people slice one piece at a time from a cake, however, they cut the slices too large, says Garner. So instead of cutting one piece at a time, slice the cake or pie into exactly the number of portions that the package indicates and then remove your slice.

Wash down cake with coffee. Coupling a dessert with a flavored coffee, which adds only about 10 calories, can bring your meal to a very satisfying close.

Freeze away temptation. You want to eat just one small serving of dessert a day, especially if you've chosen the most fattening of desserts as your passion food. At home, remove the temptation of eating more than your share by cutting your daily allotment and then storing

---

Q & A

"Emotional" Foods: Who Eats What?

Women sometimes indulge in chocolate because they feel lonely or sad. If you're looking for the perfect mood food, chocolate fills the bill. Like all melt-in-the-mouth, high-carbohydrate foods, chocolate is both soothing and stimulating. The active chemical compounds in chocolate can actually improve your mood. On top of that, chocolate causes your brain to produce the same feel-good chemicals it produces when you're in love.

Men have their own addictions. If a man eats in response to an emotion, it's anger that is most likely the trigger. Meat is the perfect mood food for working out anger or frustration because it takes effort to chew. Guys are going to want a couple of cheeseburgers or (even better) a big, juicy steak that they can really sink their teeth into. When you chomp down on food like that, your jaw is tight. Unlike chocolate, which melts passively in your mouth, meat has to be chewed aggressively.

When women feel anger or other strong emotions, they also feel the need for something really chewy. It may not be meat, although they sometimes crave that, too, but certainly something crunchy like crackers, chips, cookies, or nuts.

Expert consulted: Susan Olson, Ph.D., clinical psychologist and weight-management consultant, Seattle

the rest in the freezer. That way, the food isn't as readily available to eat.

Resisting Temptation

Sometimes, you'll be tempted to eat way more chocolate chip cookies than your eating plan could ever call for. Here are some ways to help you avoid overindulging.

Shroud the Godiva chocolates. You bought them for company, but you're contemplating eating a few, then probably a few more. Instead, put the box in a brown paper bag. When a study team headed by Maria Simonson, Sc.D., Ph.D., professor emeritus and director of the health, weight, and stress clinic at the Johns Hopkins Medical Institutions in Baltimore, put all of the doughnuts on a coffee cart in brown paper bags, the rate of purchase by factory workers fell by 50 percent. What works for doughnuts should work for chocolate.

Post it to yourself. If you often eat dessert late at night and you want to kick the habit, stick some notes to your refrigerator door. Here are some ideas.

- Closed for the evening.
- Breakfast comes soon.
- Drink ice water.
- Have a mint.
- Toothpaste your palate.
- Walk around the block.
- Are you really hungry, or just bored?

Save dessert for later. If you're an evening snacker and you usually eat dessert at dinner, Dr. Simonson advises saving the dessert for later. Gradually cut back on the size of the portion and eat it early in the evening.

Charm your mouth. Avoid having your dessert late at night, because the calories will slowly make their way to your thighs while you sleep. So if you are a 10 o'clock snacker, suck on a mint or fruit-flavored candy instead of opting for cookies, says Dr. Simonson. "It helps alleviate the need for something to chew and taste," she says. If you want something to sip late at night, Dr. Simonson recommends ice water. "It can fill you up and eliminate your craving. Many people always keep a glass of ice water by the bed." Or try low-fat or fat-free milk, she says.

Make up for it tomorrow. So it's your birthday. Someone cuts you the largest piece of cake you've ever seen, and you eat it. Don't get discouraged. Just put in some extra time exercising that week, says Garner.

Be Beverage Smart

Water. About 70 percent of the world's surface is covered by it. It makes up almost 65 percent of your body's total weight. It's pretty much everywhere but in our glasses. Given a choice between a plain glass of water and soda or fruit juice, most of us will choose soda or fruit juice.

If you want to drop a few pounds, water can be your new best friend. It's far too easy to consume a lot of calories from other beverages. A 12-ounce can of regular cola, for instance, has about 150 calories. Besides calories, other diet saboteurs lurk inside the festive-looking containers of fruit juices, sodas, and wine coolers—saboteurs such as caffeine, high-fructose corn syrup (sometimes labeled "fruit sugar"), and alcohol. So your choice of beverages can sometimes pack on as many pounds as your favorite ice cream.

Wet Your Whistle with Water

Water is, without a doubt, the best beverage choice for losing weight. It's not only fat- and calorie-free but also a way to help you eat less. Here's why.

You'll feel full. "If you drink water or have a bowl of broth-based soup before a meal, it takes up the space in your stomach that you would otherwise fill with food," says Felicia Busch, R.D., spokesperson for the American Dietetic Association. Research shows, she says, that filling up on liquids decreases the number of calories you eat in a meal.

You'll burn more calories. Drinking enough water helps your body operate under optimal conditions and may help you perform at peak metabolism. This in turn means that you may be better able to burn off fat. Drinking ice water burns a few more calories because your body heats the water to its own temperature.

Your hands and mouth are busy. If your hands and mouth are already occupied, you're less likely to eat. This trick works well at parties, where people congregate around the buffet table while stuffing themselves with hors d'oeuvres. If you have a glass of water, you can sip, not eat.

Get Your Fill of H$_2$O

Camels can go for long periods of time without water, but people can't. Water is an important part of every cell in your body, and it acts as the base in which all chemical reactions, like digestion, take place. It also plays a significant role in regulating your body temperature. So it's important to drink adequate amounts every day. "People who want to lose weight should drink more than 64 ounces of water a day," Busch says. She recommends drinking 4½ ounces of water for every 10 pounds of body weight. Thus, a 150-pound person should drink almost 68 ounces of water. That's more than a ½-gallon a day. Does that seem a little hard to swallow? Here's how to make water more appetizing and get your daily quota.

Buy bottled. If tap water doesn't appeal to your taste-buds, buy bottled water, suggests Busch. Drinking water that's already measured in bottles also makes it easier to gauge your daily intake.

Make citrus your main squeeze. If plain water doesn't float your boat, try adding a twist of lemon or some lime juice, says Ann Dubner, R.D., a nutrition consultant in private practice in Houston.

Perk it up with fruit juice. For even more flavor, dilute a quarter of a glass of fruit juice with water, says Donna Weihofen, R.D., nutritionist at the University of Wisconsin Hospital and Clinics in Madison.

Drink all day. Keep a glass of water nearby all day and take a sip every 15 minutes. "You'll be surprised by how you can end up drinking a quart of water throughout the day without even realizing it," says Dubner. And if you prefer cold water, simply fill a water bottle halfway and put it in the freezer overnight. The ice should provide cool water all day long as you refill your bottle.

Drink before you eat. Drinking a glass or two of water before meals helps take the edge off hunger so you eat less, says Dubner. Also, since many people mistake thirst for hunger, try having a glass of water the next time you want to snack.

The Diet Soda Myth

Diet soda has no calories, just like water. And it tastes better. So it should be right up there with water as a great fat-fighting beverage, right?

Not quite. Researchers at the Centre for Human Nutrition in Sheffield, England, found that people who drink beverages loaded with artificial sweeteners such as aspartame may actually eat more food. Researchers compared the food intakes of women who drank slightly less than four soda

What You Get in Latte Land

Going from plain, ordinary coffee to gourmet renditions has taken us from 10 calories and no fat per brew to as much as 300 calories and 21 grams of fat.

Here's what you get in the popular upscale drinks. (The following information comes from Starbucks; the nutrition information is based on a 12-ounce, "tall" serving.)

Caffè latte. A shot of espresso mixed with warm milk and ½ inch of foamed milk

- With whole milk: 210 calories and 11 grams of fat
- With 2% milk: 170 calories and 6 grams of fat
- With fat-free milk: 120 calories and less than a gram of fat

Caffè mocha. A shot of espresso mixed with 1½ ounces of chocolate, warm milk, and whipped cream

- With whole milk: 340 calories and 21 grams of fat
- With 2% milk: 300 calories and 16 grams of fat

cans' worth of aspartame-sweetened lemonade over the course of a day with those of women who drank the same amount of sugar-sweetened lemonade. The women who had the artificially sweetened lemonade ate more during the day following the test than those who had regular lemonade.

As for caffeine-containing sodas, caffeine makes you hungry by lowering your blood sugar, and it causes thirst by increasing your urine output. "Drinks loaded with caffeine are pretty much nutritionally worthless," says Busch, "so the less you drink of them, the better."

If you must drink diet soda, however, don't drink any more than two diet beverages a day, Dubner says.

- With fat-free milk: 260 calories and 12 grams of fat
- With whole milk, no whipped cream: 260 calories and 12 grams of fat
- With 2% milk, no whipped cream: 220 calories and 7 grams of fat
- With fat-free milk, no whipped cream: 180 calories and 3 grams of fat

Cappuccino. A shot of espresso, steamed milk, and foamed milk

- With whole milk: 140 calories and 7 grams of fat
- With 2% milk: 110 calories and 4 grams of fat
- With fat-free milk: 80 calories and less than a gram of fat

Coffee, Fat, and Calories

African tribal warriors first used ground coffee beans mixed with fat to heighten aggressiveness before going into battle. Like other caffeinated beverages, coffee makes you feel hungrier and thirstier. Plus, after a caffeine rush, you may feel tired and less able to make wise food choices.

Caffeine aside, coffee drinks are often harmful to weight-loss efforts because of what we add to them. A plain cup of coffee has between 5 and 15 calories and no fat. While we may not be as bad as the African warriors who mixed fat with their coffee beans, we come close with the cream, half-and-half, whipped cream, chocolate, honey, and almost anything else that we put in coffee. One cup of Irish coffee, for instance, has more calories than a slice of chocolate cream pie. And adding 2 tablespoons of light cream to a cup of coffee increases the calories to 59 grams and the fat to about 6 grams.

Here are a few guidelines to help you make sure those cups don't go straight to your hips or cause other health-related problems.

Drink no more than two cups a day, tops. "Sometimes, when people drink too much coffee, they feel that they need to eat something to settle their stomachs," says Christina Stark, R.D., nutrition specialist at Cornell University in

Deceptive Drinking

Few calorie counters are surprised to learn that a cheeseburger has 359 calories or a shake 340 calories. Yet they may be astonished to learn that a bottle of their favorite beverage can contain nearly as many calories.

Why do otherwise-savvy dieters get duped? Because many containers hold two or more servings, and beverage labels often list the calorie content for only one serving, which is usually 8 ounces.

Here are the calorie totals for some of the most popular beverages—the whole bottle, not just 8 ounces.

Drink	Portion (oz)	Calories
McDonald's shake (chocolate, vanilla, or strawberry)	14	340
Ocean Spray cran-grape	16	340
Nantucket Nectars cranberry juice	17.5	328

Ithaca, New York. Caffeine stimulates stomach acid secretion in some people, which can cause nausea and stomachaches.

Lighten up the lighteners. Instead of adding whole milk, cream, or half-and-half to your coffee, opt for fat-free, 1%, or 2% milk. Replacing whole milk with fat-free saves 7 to 11 grams of fat.

Try flavored beans. Using fruit-, vanilla-, or dessert-flavored coffee may be a good way to get added flavor without calories or fat.

Spice it up. For great taste without added calories or fat, dust your coffee with cinnamon.

Break the pastry connection. Some people make it a habit to have their coffee along with something fattening

Drink	Portion (oz)	Calories
Coca-Cola	20	250
Fruitopia Strawberry Passion Awareness	16	240
Snapple kiwi strawberry cocktail	16	220
Bartles and Jaymes original wine cooler	12	200
Snapple lemon iced tea	16	200
Special Recipe Natural Brew draft root beer	12	180
Mug cream soda	12	170
Arizona Iced Coffee	16	220
Beer	12	146
R. W. Knudsen Black Cherry Spritzer	10	145

such as crumb cake or doughnuts, says Stark. If coffee is your cue to reach for the baked goods, she says, you have to find a way to disassociate coffee and food. In this case, switching to decaf may not help.

"Start by substituting a low-fat treat, such as graham crackers, for the piece of pie or cake that you would normally have," says Elizabeth Brown, R.D., nutritionist and weight-control specialist at the Lehigh Valley Hospital Center for Health Promotion and Disease Prevention in Allentown, Pennsylvania. Then try to gradually wean yourself from the habit of having an accompanying treat. Adding a little milk or cinnamon to your coffee might help you to think of it as dessert so you'll still feel satisfied, she says.

Give Alcohol the Gate

Trying to save calories by skipping lunch so that you can indulge at happy hour doesn't work (although many try that strategy). Studies show that very few people decrease their food intakes when they drink alcohol. It's easy to drink many more calories than you would ever consciously consume from food, and high-fat bar food, such as peanuts, nachos, and Buffalo wings, does little to help the diet cause.

Second, as you probably could guess by the way your mouth feels the morning after, alcohol dehydrates you. So you can't count alcoholic drinks as part of your daily liquid intake, Busch says. Instead, you'll need to drink even more water to counteract each alcoholic drink you down. No one knows how much, though, as there haven't been any studies yet, she says.

If you don't drink, count yourself ahead of the game. If you decide to indulge, these tips can help you make the best choices for your waistline.

Go with one. Don't exceed one standard serving of alcohol a day. You can take your pick of either a 12-ounce beer, 1½ ounces of hard liquor, or 5 ounces of wine. If you enjoy an occasional drink, you can still have it without doing too much damage to your diet.

Begin with a virgin. Since we often gulp down our first drink, start with a nonalcoholic beverage, says Natalie Payne, R.D., nutritionist at the Washington Cancer Institute and Washington Hospital Center in Washington, D.C. Then, when the lower-calorie drink begins to fill you up, have your alcoholic beverage.

Big is better. Order a tall glass with more mixer. The bartender can then dilute the high-calorie alcohol with more club soda or diet ginger ale. Also, the larger drink will last longer, so you may not be as likely to order a second, says Weihofen.

Ask for a lower proof. Here's a simple rule: The higher the proof, the more calories it contains. So for weight watchers, it makes sense to order the brand of liquor with the lowest proof, Payne says.

Make it fat-free. If you like drinks such as white Russians or Kahlúa and creams, ask for fat-free milk, not whole milk, as the base, Payne says.

Go halvesies. For drinks made with a shot of alcohol and club soda or seltzer, get a half-shot of the alcohol and more seltzer to reduce the calories, says Payne. Be careful, though, that the bartender doesn't use a high-calorie mixer like 7Up.

The Truth about Fruit Juice

What do glasses of orange juice, cranberry juice, and grapefruit juice have in common? (a) They all have tons of vitamin C. (b) They're good for your health. (c) They can make you fat.

The answer: All of the above.

Some fruit juices have more calories than soda. A 17½-ounce bottle of Nantucket Nectars cranberry juice has more than 300 calories, while a 12-ounce can of soda has about 150. Many fruit juices contain high-fructose (fruit sugar) corn syrup. Look for 100 percent fruit juices, which are unsweetened and better choices than soda because they have nutrients, Busch says. And unlike soda, you can reduce the calories from fruit juice. Here's how to do it.

Water it down. You can easily make fruit juice a diet drink by adding more water to it, Busch says. In fact, diluted fruit juice doubles as a great low-calorie sports drink. If you're making juice from concentrate, try making two pitchers of juice from one can of concentrate. You'll cut your calories in half, and you'll get more for your money. If you like the fizz of carbonated drinks, another alternative is to make juice with sparkling water instead of tap water, Weihofen says.

Swilling Secrets

As you venture out in pursuit of beverage variety, these additional guidelines may help you make smart choices.

Milk does a diet good. If late-night eating is your down-fall, you might want to try drinking a glass of 2%, 1%, or fat-free milk instead of eating, says Maria Simonson, Sc.D., Ph.D, professor emeritus and director of the health, weight, and stress clinic at the Johns Hopkins Medical Institutions in Baltimore. It's a good low-fat alternative to the cake, cookies, or other treats you might otherwise consume.

Check the label. Although some people believe that any clear beverage is good for you, "white doesn't make it right," says Busch. Many clear beverages sold as sparkling or flavored water are really sodas in disguise. So read the labels to make sure there are no added calories.

Holiday Helpings

It's easy to gain 5 to 7 pounds between Thanksgiving and New Year's. But if you had to guess when we are most likely to put on those pounds, would you pick (a) Thanksgiving dinner, (b) Christmas dinner, (c) Hanukkah celebrations, (d) all of the above, (e) none of the above.

The answer is none of the above. "It's not one meal that adds the 5 to 7 pounds that you pick up during the holidays," says Denise T. Garner, R.D., instructor of nutrition at York College in Pennsylvania. "It's all of that extra nibbling day after day."

For many, this nibbling starts as early as Halloween, when there are often tons of candy at home and at work, says Garner.

"There's more access to food around holidays; it tends to be a very social time," says Ronna Kabatznick, Ph.D., psychologist and consultant to *Weight Watchers* magazine and founder and director of Dieters Feed the Hungry, a group in Berkeley, California, that tries to refocus dieters' attention from themselves to helping others. "Neighbors invite you for drinks, family members invite you to dinner, coworkers invite you to office parties, and there's candy on people's desks at work. These ongoing food temptations make it much harder to stick to your regular eating habits," she says.

Party Training

You can avoid that slow, steady holiday weight gain while still having a good time. Here's how to participate in the party atmosphere without gaining weight.

Don't starve ahead. Many of us skip a few meals to leave room for a big eating event. While your appetite may be stronger, your enjoyment of the experience won't be improved. "By dinner, you'll be starving, so you won't make good decisions about what you eat," says Barbara Whedon, R.D., a dietitian at Thomas Jefferson University Hospital in Philadelphia.

Load up with lean before the party. Instead of cutting back on meals before a big holiday event, appease your appetite with some low-fat food beforehand. "If you curb your appetite, you can make better choices," says Whedon. Some good pre-party fare includes soup or a few pieces of fruit. By taking in at least some calories before the big event, you take the edge off your appetite and help keep yourself from going overboard.

Pick just four. Whether it's hors d'oeuvres or desserts, limit yourself to four samplings, says Garner. That means fresh vegetables with 1 tablespoon of dip, one spinach ball, one mini egg roll, and one cube of cheese. For dessert, you can have a taste of pecan pie, one forkful of cheesecake, a bite of fudge, and one cookie. If you feel awkward taking such small portions, give the rest to a friend. This way, you can taste the four foods you really want without loading up on calories.

Talk more. The more you talk, the less you eat, says Garner.

Don't have a white Christmas. Lay off the eggnog. One 8-ounce glass runs about 342 calories and has 19 grams of fat, which makes it a lot like melted ice cream. Hot spiced cider is a better bet; it's fat-free and just as festive.

Begin with the buffet. While this is usually where a party's heartiest and heaviest fare resides, you should be able to scavenge at least a few good-tasting items that don't contain fat in the double digits. "Some good choices are things like shrimp cocktail, fruit salad, and any vegetable that's light on the dip," Whedon says. A large steamed shrimp has only about 5 calories, with just a trace of fat. You can even have some cocktail sauce, at 45 calories per tablespoon. And don't forget the pretzels, which are also low in fat.

"If there's a cold-cut platter, stick with turkey or lean roast beef," Whedon adds. By contrast, other meats, such as bologna, salami, and pepperoni, and most cheeses are extremely high in fat.

Favor the hostess with something fat-free. Take a light alternative, such as a vegetable platter or fruit plate, to the party. Even nonalcoholic beer or sparkling grape juice makes a nice offering. These make warm and generous gifts to the hostess, and they give you something to nibble on or sip that won't make you feel guilty.

Give temptations the brush-off. After you've had a few hors d'oeuvres, sneak off to the bathroom and brush your teeth. You'll be less likely to eat more cocktail wieners if you know they're going to taste like spearmint.

Pass on the plate. Instead, opt for a dainty cocktail napkin. Carry your finger foods one small portion at a time, and that's how you'll eat.

Or use a fork. When at holiday parties, you really should be wary of most finger foods. The best foods to eat with your hands are shrimp, vegetables, and fruits.

Use your other hand. This is a surprisingly effective and simple trick that works well at any party where finger foods are a fixture. Keep your drink in your dominant hand so that if you do reach for a snack, you'll have to think about it a bit more than usual.

Learn to say no. Do you have trouble turning down another serving of deep-fried cheese balls? Here are some polite-yet-firm responses to the persuasive entreaty "Have some more. . . . I made it just for you."

- "No, thank you."
- "I'm full."
- "I appreciate all of your effort, and I've enjoyed every bite."
- "If you want to give me more, I can take another portion home."

"If you keep saying no, the person doing the coaxing will soon lose their power over you," says Dr. Kabatznick. When all else fails, use the medical excuse. "Many people with serious weight problems tell me that the only way they've ever gotten people to stop pushing food is by saying that they have an allergy or that they're concerned about their cholesterol or that their doctor advises against something," says Ronette Kolotkin, Ph.D., director of the behavioral program at the Duke University Diet and Fitness Center in Durham, North Carolina, and coauthor of *The Duke University Medical Center Book of Diet and Fitness.*

Always keep something on your plate. During the holiday season, an empty plate tells the host that you are hungry for more. "No one believes you're full if your plate is empty. But if your plate still has a bit of food on it, that sends the signal that you've had all you can possibly eat," says Whedon. Make sure what you leave behind is your least favorite dish. Otherwise, you might eat it, thus devouring your anti-fat shield.

Tighten your belt. Wearing something snug to the party can serve as a restraining device for your stomach, says

Mindy Hermann, R.D., a nutrition counselor in Mount Kisco, New York.

Keep your hands full of anything but food. Baby pictures, a sprig of mistletoe, and a camera are all good items to take with you to holiday gatherings where food is the focus.

Visualize. "When you do a mental dress rehearsal, it's like going through the experience, so when you actually experience the event, it's easier, and you make better choices because you've already practiced them," says Judy E. Marshel, R.D., director of Health Resources in Great Neck, New York, and former senior nutritionist for Weight Watchers International.

Less Holiday Nibbling

Many of the extra calories that we swallow over the holidays are eaten unconsciously. As we bake, we may sample the dough. We try free samples at the grocery store. We have a slice of pizza at the mall while shopping for Christmas gifts. And we have a few too many cookies everywhere we go. Here's how to keep those calories from turning into pounds.

Bake in the morning. You'll be less likely to sample dough, nuts, and chocolate chips just after breakfast than in the afternoon or evening, says Garner. Another good trick is to chew gum while you bake.

Practice sweat equity. Keeping up with your exercise program during the cold, dark winter months will go a long way toward keeping off winter weight gain, and it will help to control holiday stress as well. Do aerobics to cable exercise shows, get an exercise bike, or join a gym.

You can even be active on the actual holiday. "If you're spending the holiday with children, consider going sledding or ice-skating; these are non-food-centered ways of spending time. If you're with adults, go hiking or visit a museum," says Dr. Kabatznick.

"Exercise is the best single thing you can do during the holidays," Dr. Kabatznick adds. "It's a tension reliever, plus it gives you food credits so you can overindulge a bit. Swim extra laps. Walk an extra mile or two a day. Enjoy your body in ways that don't have to do with food."

Eat before you mall. If you fill up before you shop for gifts, you'll be less likely to munch on sweet rolls, slurp shakes, and contemplate a plate of nachos.

Don't cook on empty. You know that grocery shopping when you're hungry is a no-no. The same advice applies to cooking holiday dinners. If you're hungry and you surround yourself with food, you're bound to nibble through the preparation, and you'll probably make more food than you really need. Take the edge off by having a light but satisfying snack, such as nonfat or low-fat yogurt or graham crackers, before you begin to cook.

Break your date with Frosty. And don't hang out with the Grinch, Jimmy Stewart, or Charlie Brown either since such TV dates are usually accompanied by bowls and bowls of couch-potato food. Instead, get on your stationary bike and ride from Nazareth to Bethlehem (about 70 miles as the dove flies) over the 12 days of Christmas. Or play holiday tunes on your headset while you exercise. If you just can't drag yourself away from that favorite holiday rerun, replace the snacks on your lap with those holiday cards that you've been meaning to address.

No More Stuffing Yourself Silly

Why don't we gain extra weight around summer holidays, like Independence Day, Memorial Day, and Labor Day?

Because we're outside cycling, walking on the beach, tossing horseshoes, and playing tag with the kids. We're burning more calories, and we're not eating as many of them. A typical cookout menu of grilled chicken, pasta salad, and watermelon doesn't pack quite the same fat-and-calorie punch as typical Thanksgiving, Christmas, or New Year's fare, says Garner. But you can keep those three winter feasts from turning into body fat. Here's how.

Eat the chow, free the fat. While not all holiday calories can be easily trimmed away, you can limit the damage. If you're eating turkey, for example, a serving of white meat has less than half the fat of a comparable serving of dark meat. If you're having a roast, trim away the visible fat, including the crispy bits; they're burned fat, but they're still fat.

Be careful with add-ons. Don't cover your plate with a whopping serving of stuffing and a pool of gravy. Both gravy and stuffing are often made with butter or meat drippings, which are extremely fattening.

Create borders. As you fill your plate for a holiday feast, maintain a little margin of space between portions of food—just enough room so that you can still see some plate. The result is that you'll automatically keep portions to a more reasonable size. A plate with 7 ounces of turkey, 2 cups of stuffing, 4 ounces of gravy, 1 cup of candied sweet potatoes, ½ cup of cranberry sauce, and 1 cup of green beans all smashed against one another with no space to breathe would come to 1,422 calories. The same foods on the same-size plate, but with portions cut in half to allow for space between the foods, would amount to only 711 calories.

Take off the turkey's coat. Without the skin, a 3½-ounce serving of white turkey meat has only 157 calories, with 18 percent of that from fat. Dark meat is fattier: A 3½-ounce skinless serving has 187 calories, with 35 percent from fat. The same-size serving of white meat with skin has 197 calories, with 38 percent of that from fat; dark meat with skin has 221 calories, with 46 percent from fat. So as long as you skip the skin, you'll do fine.

Say yes to yams. Canned candied yams have only 240 calories per 4-ounce serving, and many brands have no fat. Check the label to be sure. Adding butter to canned or fresh yams made at home obviously adds calories and fat.

Add a twist to holiday baking. Make lower-fat meringue cookies or gingersnaps instead of chocolate chip or butter cookies.

Be selective. When you think about it, many of the foods that we enjoy at holiday time, such as roast turkey, sweet potatoes, and apple cider, are perfectly healthful when prepared simply and eaten in reasonable quantities, points out Marshel. Focus on the peas, broccoli, and lean meat; go easy on the gravy, butter, au gratin dishes, and pie.

Take it and leave it. Chances are, there's so much going on at the dinner table that few people will really notice what you have or haven't eaten. So if what you do or do not put on your plate becomes an issue, just take what's served. "If worse comes to worst, you can take the food and not eat it," says Dr. Kabatznick.

Have dessert for dinner. Most holiday meals are eaten between the normal lunch and dinner hours. So there's no real reason to have another full-fledged meal around 7:00 P.M. Instead, save your dessert for that time, suggests Garner.

Practice recovery. What happens if you go completely AWOL from your fat-fighting plan? The trick to emerging from the holiday food fest without permanently losing your weight-loss motivation is to accept the fact that you've slipped a bit and then get on with your wholesome new way of low-fat living. Immediately resume your usual food-and-fitness program, no matter how many days you've been away from it.

Help Yourself to Better Holiday Cuisine

Even just one helping of a typical Thanksgiving dinner can pack more than 1,000 calories and 50 grams of fat. (Just imagine the big fat damage when you eat seconds or thirds!) Yet you can slash half of those calories and fat grams from holiday meals and still eat your favorite festive foods.

"Decide what food is most important to you or what food is eaten or available only during that particular holiday season, and enjoy a moderate amount," says Mary Pat Bolton, R.D., lead nutritionist for the Women's Health Initiative at Baylor College of Medicine in Houston.

There are also easy cooking strategies to remove fat and calories from your typical holiday fare without sacrificing flavor. Here's a holiday-by-holiday breakdown of some fat- and calorie-slashing secrets.

Thanksgiving: Traditional

- Five ounces of roasted turkey, white and dark meat, with skin (291 calories and 14 grams of fat)
- 1 cup of bread stuffing made from a mix (356 calories and 7 grams of fat)
- One slice (⅛ of a 9-inch pie) of homemade pumpkin pie (316 calories and 14 grams of fat)

Thanksgiving: Slimmed Down

- 5 ounces of turkey breast without skin (238 calories and 7 grams of fat)

- 1 cup of cornbread stuffing made outside the bird with chicken broth instead of lots of eggs and drippings (265 calories and 8 grams of fat)
- One slice of pumpkin pie made with nonfat and reduced-fat dairy products (288 calories and 8 grams of fat)

Christmas: Traditional

- 6 ounces of boneless cured ham (303 calories and 15 grams of fat)
- 1 cup of mashed potatoes made with whole milk and butter (223 calories and 9 grams of fat)
- Three homemade sugar cookies (198 calories and 10 grams of fat)

Christmas: Slimmed Down

- 3 ounces of ham (151 calories and 8 grams of fat)
- 1 cup of mashed potatoes made with nonfat sour cream and garlic (169 calories and 2 grams of fat)
- Three gingersnaps (87 calories and 2 grams of fat)

New Year's Day: Traditional

- 8 ounces of eggnog (341 calories and 19 grams of fat)
- Six to eight nachos with cheese, beans, ground beef, and peppers (569 calories and 31 grams of fat)

New Year's Day: Slimmed Down

- 4 ounces of eggnog (171 calories and 10 grams of fat). After you've had your eggnog, stick with sparkling water (0 calories and 0 grams of fat), or have a cup of hot mulled cider made by simmering 6 cups of apple cider, one cinnamon stick, three whole cloves, three allspice berries, and strips of orange rind in a saucepan over medium heat for 10 to 15 minutes. Strain before serving. This makes 6 cups (63 calories and 0 grams of fat per cup)

- Homemade nachos made by cutting 12 corn tortillas into quarters and topping them with low-fat Monterey Jack cheese, salsa, beans, and peppers (hold the beef). This makes 48 nachos (351 calories and 7 grams of fat per 12 chips)

Valentine's Day: Traditional

- 1½-ounce chocolate bar (207 calories and 14 grams of fat)

Valentine's Day: Slimmed Down

- ½ cup of strawberry frozen yogurt with 2 tablespoons of chocolate syrup drizzled over it (192 calories and 3 grams of fat)

Easter: Traditional

- A basket of chocolate bunnies and eggs (143 calories and 10 grams of fat per ounce; for 10 1-ounce bunnies and eggs, 1,430 calories and 100 grams of fat)
- 5 ounces of roasted leg of lamb with ½ cup of steamed asparagus and ½ cup of boiled potatoes (456 calories and 23 grams of fat)

Easter: Slimmed Down

- A 1-ounce chocolate treat per basket, with the rest of the space filled with jelly beans (104 calories and a trace of fat per ounce of jelly beans (about 10); for 1 ounce of chocolate plus 50 jelly beans, 663 calories and 10 grams of fat)

- 3 ounces of lamb with 1 cup of steamed asparagus and 1 cup of boiled potatoes (399 calories and 15 grams of fat)

Memorial or Labor Day: Traditional

- Two pieces (about 6 ounces total) of cold fast-food fried chicken, white meat from the breast or wing (494 calories and 30 grams of fat)
- 1 cup of potato salad (358 calories and 21 grams of fat)
- 1 cup of baked beans (382 calories and 13 grams of fat)
- One 3-inch-square packaged brownie (227 calories and 9 grams of fat)

Memorial or Labor Day: Slimmed Down

- Two pieces (about 8 ounces total) of cold chicken breast without the skin, baked without oil (318 calories and 8 grams of fat)
- 1 cup of potato or pasta salad made with fat-free mayonnaise (304 calories and 5 grams of fat)
- 1 cup of low-fat vegetarian baked beans (236 calories and 1 gram of fat) or 1 cup of low-fat nonvegetarian baked beans made with low-fat turkey sausage and reduced-sodium chicken broth (272 calories and 2 grams of fat)
- One wedge of watermelon (92 calories and 1 gram of fat)

Fourth of July: Traditional

- A 5-ounce grilled hamburger (426 calories and 23 grams of fat)
- A 3-ounce grilled Italian sausage (268 calories and 21 grams of fat)

Fourth of July: Slimmed Down

- A 5-ounce grilled turkey burger made with lean ground turkey, minced onions, garlic, red peppers, celery, and a small amount of tomato paste (289 calories and 3 grams of fat); you can add lots of nearly fat-free toppings such as tomatoes, lettuce, pepper rings, and onions
- One-half (about 3 ounces) grilled skinless chicken breast (142 calories and 3 grams of fat)

Strategies
for Special Situations

When it comes to sticking to a weight-loss plan, not all people are created equal. Some of us have incredible demands on our time, making regular exercise difficult to fit in. Others have a harder time resisting food, mainly because it seems to be ever present. Some of us have careers that require us to eat out nearly every day. And still others work such odd hours that breakfast becomes dinner and dinner becomes breakfast.

Considering the differences in lifestyle, it's no wonder that a reduced-calorie eating plan may work for some people but not others. Similarly, while some weight-loss tips could change your life forever, they could be no help at all to someone else.

So when it comes right down to it, each of us must in part design an eating plan that fits her personal lifestyle, says Kristine Napier, R.D., author of *Eat to Heal*. Napier identified the most common types of people who struggle with weight. Here, she offers the most up-to-date, realistic, and beneficial advice on how to modify a fat-fighting plan to fit your lifestyle.

Midlife Crash Dieters

You may have developed the weight-loss technique way back in high school. You went out with some friends. You finished off half a pizza. You downed the largest hot fudge sundae the ice cream shop could make. And then you felt fat.

So you didn't eat anything the next day. At the end of the day, you happily looked down at your flat belly and the gap between your waist and your jeans, and you knew that fasting for a day did the job. So crash dieting became the norm for you.

The problem is, sometime during your thirties, the technique stopped working as well. In your forties, it doesn't seem to work at all, at least not permanently. No matter what diet you try, from cabbage soup to eating nothing at all, you lose only a few pounds and then gain back more. As soon as you splurge on an evening of appetizers, wine, pizza, and one double-dip ice cream cone, you gain 2 pounds. And sipping mineral water and eating salads for a few days doesn't seem to get rid of the weight the way it used to.

It's time to get off the calorie roller coaster. You need to take a challenging but important step: Start eating real food in realistic amounts. That's hard for chronic crash dieters, who are used to eating what they consider "forbidden" foods and then later purging themselves of the damage with intense exercise, starvation, or a combination of the two. Here are some solutions.

Consult a nutrition savant. If you can, consult a registered dietitian to help you determine how many calories you need to eat to maintain or lose weight, based on your body size and activity level. You'll probably be surprised at how much food you actually should be eating. And having a dietitian tell you so will help cement your trust in this new eating lifestyle. Don't be tempted to resume your past vicious cycle, which gradually helped you pick up an extra 30 or so pounds.

Find portion control. You need to meticulously measure food and discover healthy portion sizes. That way, you'll never feel overloaded and as if you were going to burst, or so empty that your stomach growls. Plan to include a favorite food in a healthy portion daily, preferably early in the day, to help you stick to your eating plan.

Eat breakfast. You're probably used to skimping on breakfast in an attempt to cut calories. But starting the day with an energy-packed meal will keep you satisfied through the morning as well as boost your job performance. Most important, you'll eat less later in the day.

Satisfy snack attacks. Plan two snacks each day that satisfy your tastebuds as well as your hunger. Don't make the mistake of talking yourself into something like carrots when you really crave chocolate chip cookies. Chances are, you'll fill up on carrots, then you'll have the cookies anyway. Instead, plan to have a snack of one chocolate chip cookie and one glass of fat-free milk in the mid-afternoon. In the long run, you'll eat fewer calories.

Have a real dinner. Do you usually prepare a big meal for the family but make yourself a salad to save calories? Such deprivation only leads to binge eating later on. Eat a regular dinner with your family.

Living with Others Who Eat Heartily

How can you feed others the incredible number of calories they seem to need without gaining weight yourself and without cooking two entirely different meals?

Plan, plan, plan. You can eat the same foods as others as long as you cook lower-fat meals and dish out a smaller helping for yourself than you do for them. They can serve themselves in more generous double or triple portions. Plan menus carefully to make sure that you cook fat-fighting foods. You will not only be fighting fat yourself, but you will also be doing others a favor, reducing their risks of heart disease and other conditions associated with high-fat diets. Try roasting a chicken with new potatoes, carrots, onions, and brussels sprouts, for example, for a low-fat meal that also provides plenty of nutrition.

Study portion sizes carefully. Measure portions a few times and then periodically check on your ability to eye-ball them.

Put margarine or butter on the table, not on the food. You can opt not to add any to your food while others use it.

Buy things you don't like. When it comes to snacks, you have a couple of options, depending on your willpower. If your willpower is of stellar quality, buy snacks for your family that you'll declare off-limits to yourself. (Don't go overboard, though, with items that aren't very nutritious or that are heavily laden with fat, especially saturated fat.) If, on the other hand, your willpower is less than mighty, you could at least consider purchasing things you don't like. They love fig bars and you hate them? Great! Fig bars are a nutritious snack, anyway, so you'll be doing the others a favor. Nacho cheese–flavored tortilla chips are one of your downfalls? Just don't bring them into the house.

Eat vegetables. If you find yourself tempted to take second helpings along with your dining companions, try cooking yourself an extra vegetable at dinner, and make it something that you really love. Are you crazy about asparagus with freshly squeezed lemon juice? Don't hesitate to add it to the menu frequently. Or maybe baby carrots cooked with brown sugar and cinnamon strike your fancy. Whatever it is, having another vegetable to eat while others continue to chow down will keep you from helping yourself to another portion just to be sociable.

Choose desserts carefully. Tell the family that you have a new kitchen rule: Dessert will be served not nightly but on Wednesdays and Saturdays (or whatever days are convenient for you). When dessert night rolls around, serve yourself a small portion and enjoy every bite. For the rest of the week, make fresh fruit the family dessert, splurging on raspberries, strawberries, or whatever your family likes. To make it special, buy low-fat or nonfat frozen dairy toppings and serve yourself one generous dollop.

Slim down when they're not around. Make a point of eating lean when you're alone, such as at lunch. But don't starve yourself, either. Sitting down to the dinner table ravenously hungry may be your undoing. In fact, you might try having a glass of vegetable juice or fruit juice an hour or two before dinner to turn down your appetite.

Empty Nesters

As midlife approaches, many women go from having no time to themselves due to the demands of a growing family to suddenly having too much time. In addition to learning how to fill the physical and emotional voids left by departing children, "empty nest" moms must learn how to shop and cook for two (or sometimes one) in ways that will prevent weight gain.

Mothers often think about feeding their children (and husbands) as a means of not only filling their stomachs but also healing their hurts and rewarding their accomplishments. With the children gone, food often takes on a new meaning for the women; it can (at least temporarily) fill the emotional void and heal their own loneliness. In addition, it's hard to get used to making less food. If you have poured an entire box of spaghetti into a pot of boiling water for the past 15 or so years, for instance, you'll need to give yourself time to adjust to making less pasta. Here's how to make the transition.

Plan a daily menu. From that menu, make a shopping list and stick to it when you shop. This will keep you from overbuying. Are you tempted to pick up chips, cookies, and ice cream just in case the kids stop buy? Don't. You may feel obligated to eat them just to get rid of them.

Stash the money you save on groceries. Watch it grow, and promise to buy yourself something special with it. Having another incentive to not overbuy groceries can be a big help.

Spoil the kids when you see them. Having the kids over for dinner? Take this opportunity to make their favorite dishes, then send the leftovers home with them.

Find new interests. Do you continue to bake because you love to do it but then eat the cookies, cakes, and pies yourself? If so, find another hobby.

Go to a gym. Do you get lonely at mealtime, either because you live alone or because your husband travels frequently? Find an exercise class that meets late in the day. It will take your mind off fixing and eating a big dinner, and it may reduce your appetite.

Make your own frozen dinners. Find items that freeze so that you can make a full batch and put some away for another meal. Or at least cook something that you can warm up later in the week for a second meal. Believe it or not, you'll come to enjoy not having to cook every night.

Working Odd Hours

In nursing school, no one seemed able to keep weight on, recalls Napier. The class schedule was grueling and left little time for sleeping or eating.

Fifteen years later, the schedule doesn't seem that much

easier, but now it seems to promote weight gain instead of weight loss. The same is true of other jobs where the hours change from day to night and night to day. All-night supermarket cashiers, police officers, and others who do shift work have unique weight-related problems. Those who work odd hours seem to pick up a few pounds whenever they switch shifts. Yet changing sleep patterns alone don't generate weight gain. What's going on?

Indirectly, the fatigue that accompanies shift changes is probably to blame. Many people respond to that fatigue by eating because munching helps them stay awake. Losing track of regular mealtimes also adds calories. When you're up at odd hours, you often eat at odd times and may have four or five good-size meals without even realizing it. In addition, many workers are captive victims of vending machines or midnight cafeteria fare, neither of which is conducive to eating on the lighter side. Here's how to fight fat while surviving shift changes.

Pack your food. Pack snacks and a lunch for your shift. In addition to carrot sticks, take a fresh orange (peeled and sealed in a resealable plastic bag so that you can't use the I-don't-have-time excuse) and a sandwich with good-quality protein (like turkey on whole wheat bread) and a juicy tomato slice to make lunch interesting. Also pack a small helping of your favorite treat. Do you love chocolate because it helps you get through those interminable nights? Pack one or two small chocolate pieces such as chocolate kisses, which are about ⅕ of an ounce each.

Leave your money at home. Even if you've packed a lunch, you might not be able to resist a coworker's offer to bring you a treat from the cafeteria. So don't take money to work. To keep you out of range of the food concession, pack your own diet soft drink or sparkling water. Invest in a good Thermos so you can make gourmet coffee for yourself. If you have errands to run on the way home from work, lock whatever money you'll need in the glove compartment of the car.

Wait until you are awake to think about dinner. Plan your at-home meals carefully, too, and do it when you are not hungry or tired. Do you generally arrive home in the morning, hungry and tired, after an all-nighter? Each night before you leave for work, fix yourself a meal and then heat it in the microwave when you get home. Or set out the cooking utensils and at least some of the ingredients before you leave for work. Yet another option is to buy healthy frozen meals and heat them in the microwave.

Plan regular eating times. Develop an eating schedule for your odd hours, trying to include three small meals and one or two small snacks. Figure out when you like breakfast and then plan healthy breakfasts for those times. Ditto for lunch and dinner. Maybe you like to have your big meal while you're working. If so, take a serving of lasagna or low-fat meat loaf and a baked potato with steamed broccoli to work and heat them in the microwave, if one is available.

Don't play hooky from food. Avoid skipping meals because you are tired. You'll only make up for it later, as it will eventually make you ravenously hungry and set you up for a binge.

Don't fall into the fast-food trap. Fast food is famous for hidden calories and fat. If you have steel-reinforced willpower, however, you can occasionally stop at fast-food places and choose their lower-fat fare, such as a grilled chicken breast sandwich, fajitas, or a salad with low-fat dressing.

On-the-Job Wining and Dining

In many professions, doing business over breakfast, lunch, or dinner is routine. Many financial planners, lawyers, publicists, and others need to meet their clients when they are available, which often includes mealtime. In some professions, meeting over lunch or dinner gives you an opportunity to forge good relations by treating your companion to a nice meal.

Even if you are careful, in just 4 years at such a job, you could pick up as much as 12 pounds. Two extra teaspoons of butter per day, for example, is about 68 calories. If you work 50 weeks a year and dine out three times a week, that adds up to 10,200 calories, which in turn equals about 3 pounds a year.

You think you're being cautious: You ration the butter to just one pat on a lunchtime roll. Most nights, you hold yourself to a salad or choose grilled fish in a light sauce or a grilled chicken breast sandwich. And if you order dessert, you don't finish it.

Even so, you simply cannot account for all the hidden calories. That single pat of butter, for instance, is really nearly 2 teaspoons instead of the scant 1 you'd use at home. Then there's the "light" sauce for the grilled fish. Skillfully prepared with lemon juice and herbs, it looks and tastes low-fat, but it's usually loaded with butter and cream. And when you chose those grilled chicken breast sandwiches, you probably didn't know that the chef soaked butter into the bun (no wonder they taste so moist).

No matter how often you have to eat out, though, you can maintain your figure and fight fat. Here are some dining-out secrets.

Get to know the food servers. When you can, frequent the same restaurants and get to know the staff. If possible, arrange to speak with the chef at off-peak hours and ask what he can do to cut calories for you. Then always order the same type of food there, instructing the server to tell the chef who is requesting the food.

Don't even think about opening the menu. Once you open the menu, temptation kicks in. Instead, be committed to ordering grilled chicken, fish, or lean beef. Grilled tenderloin, for example, is very lean and often excellent tasting. Just ask the waiter or waitress to serve it without sauce.

Take some home for later. Restaurant portions are overly generous. Usually, you eat more than you need just because the food is sitting in front of you. Size up the portion when it comes (use a scale at home to really learn healthy portion sizes), take what you would for a normal, healthy-size portion, and ask the server to remove the rest or pack it up for you to take home. Rest assured, it's no longer a sign of poor manners to avoid wasting food.

Eat low-calorie foods first. Fill up on salad or a broth-based soup, and then just sample the main course you chose.

Work in some fruit. Like most people who eat out frequently, you probably don't get enough fruits and vegetables in your diet. Get into the habit of ordering a fresh fruit cup for an appetizer and fresh berries for dessert. If you'd like, order the berries with cream, but have the server give them just a dab or two.

Aim for two super-healthy meals a week. Promise yourself at least one or two meals of steamed vegetables per week. Any restaurant can do this for you. In some, you may even be able to get the chef to accent them with freshly chopped basil or another favorite herb. Planning ahead can be a huge fat saver.

Working at Home

Your friends may think you are so lucky: You have a full-time career, and you can still be at home. You can make your own hours and take breaks to get outside when the weather is beautiful.

In theory, working at home is great. But, just as with a regular office job, work-related stress makes you turn to food, which is only too available just down the hall in the kitchen. Food is just too handy, and you can always go back for more. You don't even have to search for change.

What's the answer? If you have a home-based office, you must counter several things to control excess calorie intake. You'll need to put away food reminders, define the line between home and work, and find an alternative to stress-induced eating. Here are some thoughts on how to tackle the problems.

Try not to work in the kitchen. Working all day around constant temptation is more than even the most virtuous people can handle.

Do the dishes, then start work. Before you start to work, let the answering machine take your calls, and clean up the breakfast dishes. Later, do the same with the lunch dishes. Working around food and dishes is another powerful reminder to eat.

Take a lunch break. Eat meals at a set time, away from your work. Carrying food to your desk blurs the line between work and home, making eating too accessible.

Set a time to start dinner. Leave work behind you for that specified time. Again, mixing meal preparation with work tends to let eating spill over into your work life and leads to overeating.

Prepare for dealing with stress without food. Do you have room in your home office or somewhere nearby for an exercise bike or other type of equipment? Rather than get up from your desk for a cookie when stress and frustration strike, take a 2-minute exercise break.

Stressed-Out Meal Skippers

For those with hectic schedules, eating becomes a catch-as-catch-can affair. The day begins in such a whirlwind that you usually don't have time for breakfast. For whatever reason, you also end up skipping lunch most days or you grab something on the fly from a vending machine. Having skipped the first two meals of the day, you usually eat whatever you can when you walk in the house after work, shoving things into your mouth at the speed of light. Then you're not hungry at dinner, and you only toy with your food. An hour or so later, when the junk-food fullness wears off, you ransack the kitchen for snacks.

True, you can't change your busy schedule. But you can change your response to it. Here are some suggestions.

Make breakfast at night. Pack breakfast in the evening and set it next to your purse or briefcase. A cereal bar, a banana, or an apple are great on-the-go breakfast foods.

While you're at it, make lunch too. If you're going to be away from home at lunchtime, pack something the night before that doesn't need to be refrigerated. If you're going to be home, make something—a sandwich or salad, perhaps—and pop it in the refrigerator. Having something ready takes at least some of the rush out of lunchtime and keeps you from grabbing junk food.

Make a super bowl. Each night, prepare a fruit bowl for the following day. It should have no less than one piece of fruit per family member, and at least two for you. When you walk in the door famished at the end of the day, reach for a piece of fruit, and encourage everyone else to do the same.

Fill up with liquids. As you prepare dinner, pour yourself a tall glass of sparkling water, iced tea, vegetable juice, or fruit juice. This will keep you from eating and will also hydrate you. If you've been running around all day, you probably haven't had nearly enough to drink.

Set kitchen hours. After you've fixed the next day's fruit bowl and your portable breakfast, close up the kitchen and turn off the lights. This serves as a physical reminder that food is off-limits until the next day. Even if you are hungry, the dark kitchen should turn you away and encourage you to start off the next day on the right track.

Those Who Can't Exercise

People who have a chronic condition will most likely need to modify their exercise programs. Certainly, a gentle swim may be in the cards for some, or perhaps an easy stroll. But for many, working up a sweat just might not be possible.

In addition to physical restrictions on exercise options, you may take medication that slows your metabolism or increases your appetite. Or perhaps you have no chronic ailment but are dead set against exercise for some reason. Either way, read on. The following information will work for anyone with limitations.

To slim down, you must maximize nutrient density. In other words, since there's a limit to how many calories you can burn off with physical activity, every calorie you consume must be packed with vitamins and minerals. Premium ice cream, for example, has low nutrient density: The few nutrients it contains (like protein and calcium) are accompanied by loads and loads of calories from fat and sugar. Nonfat yogurt, on the other hand, has a higher nutrient density, with 6 grams of protein in just 100 calories.

Here's another example. Strawberry shortcake isn't devoid of nutrients since the strawberries supply some vitamin C and folate, an important B vitamin. But once you pile the strawberries on the cake and hide them underneath whipped cream, those vitamins "cost" lots of calories, so the caloric cost of 50 milligrams of vitamin C in strawberry shortcake is 352 calories. In contrast, a heaping bowl of strawberries alone is extremely nutrient dense.

You harvest 50 milligrams of vitamin C, as well as folate and fiber, for just 50 calories. What's more, you have lots more calories to spend throughout the rest of the day.

Here are other ways to harvest nutrient density without sacrificing flavor.

Fashion dessert from a rainbow of fresh fruits. Combining kiwifruit with strawberries and bananas, for example, creates the explosion of flavor you're looking for and also satisfies even the sweetest sweet tooth and the most discerning tastebuds. If it's creamy texture you want, try fat-free or low-fat frozen whipped toppings.

Buy exceptionally great cuts of meat. Generally, you'll find them in the gourmet section of your grocery store's meat department. No matter what your budget, though, you'll be able to afford them because you'll be buying so much less. You'll select just 3 to 4 ounces of uncooked meat for yourself, for example, instead of the ½ pound or more that's customary. You'll harvest lots of protein, iron, vitamin B_{12}, and zinc in that lean and luscious meat.

Choose hearty, whole-grain breads. The best-tasting breads come fresh from the bakery. You can preserve bakery freshness by freezing the bread in individual portions the day you buy it. Just slice the bread (if it didn't come that way) and close it securely in resealable bags. The whole-grain goodness not only is exceptionally satisfying but also is quantum leaps more nutritious than white bread. You'll find it so satisfying that you won't need (or even want) butter or margarine on it. When you use it to make a sandwich, you'll be loading your meal with lots of minerals, B vitamins, and fiber.

Have a mixed medley. Just as you combine fruits to create a flavor explosion, you can blend many vegetables together. Accent tomatoes with sweet onions, basil, and portobello mushrooms, for example, splashing everything with flavor-loaded balsamic vinegar and just a touch of virgin olive oil. Add crunchy chopped cucumbers to leafy romaine lettuce, deliciously satisfying sweet red peppers, and smooth mushrooms in a lunchtime salad that you've also loaded with slightly nutty chickpeas. The flavor is intense, and the nutrient density can't be beat.

Have what you crave. Use some high-fat, high-calorie ingredients to lend interest and satisfaction (sometimes more psychological than physical) to your meals. But use them wisely and sparingly. Use a teaspoon of melted butter, for example, (yes, real melted butter) to top fresh fish, but first load it with plenty of sautéed fresh herbs. Fresh rosemary, for example, sautéed in a teaspoon of butter with fresh garlic, adds an absolute flavor explosion to even the driest, most boring white fish.

Stay-at-Home Moms

Children are like nonstop vacuum cleaners. Their small stomach capacities prevent them from eating enough food at one sitting to keep them full for a long time. Yet they need to eat a phenomenal number of calories to fuel their active, growing bodies, so they're constantly searching for snacks, drinks, and more snacks.

The problem is, it seems as though the more your children eat, the more weight *you* gain. You're a grown-up. You're no longer growing (at least not vertically), so you can't eat that many calories if you want to stay thin. Yet along with the kids, you're having a taste of peanut butter here, half of a cookie there, and maybe a glass of juice several times throughout the day. And then there are the last bites of food you clean up after you've already eaten your share. If little Marissa leaves a clump of macaroni and cheese and pint-size Tommy stops eating with a third of his hot dog to go, you end up finishing their meals. It may not seem like a lot of caloric damage, but it adds up.

Let's tally up those last few bites. The last little bit of hot dog, for instance, has about 80 calories, and the last few spoonfuls of macaroni and cheese about 100 calories. If you ate just that much extra food a day, you'd gain a pound in 20 weeks and somewhere around 12 pounds in 5 years. Just ½ cup of apple juice (most adults drink more) adds another 60 calories, and an extra cookie packs 50 to 100 calories. It's easy to understand, then, how weight creeps on with all of those extra "bites."

To counteract this weight gain, you first need to distinguish between "parent" food and "kiddie" food. By design, children's foods pack a lot of calories for their punch. That's because kids need to stuff their tiny stomachs with those calories so they can grow. As adults, though, we need to do the opposite—feel satisfied on relatively fewer calories. So, even if it seems that you're wasting food, you'll want to incorporate the following into your fat-fighting plan.

Picture a garbage disposal. You can even put a picture of one on your refrigerator. Tell yourself that that's where leftover food should go, not in your stomach.

Eat adult food. Make yourself a gorgeous salad while the kids are eating lunch, with several vegetables and a good source of lean protein such as lean ham, chickpeas, reduced-fat cheese, tuna, or leftover roast chicken. Once you put the kids down for their afternoon naps, settle down with classical music playing, a goblet full of sparkling water, and your salad set on a pretty place mat. You'll feel special and satisfied.

Switch to better snack food. Start your children's healthy eating habits early. Instead of double-fudge cookies, offer them simpler shortbread cookies. Or try apple slices, a banana, popcorn, or yogurt. These are things that you can snack on, too, without breaking your calorie budget.

Set eating hours. Open the kitchen just twice, once in the morning and once in the afternoon, for planned snacks rather than let the kids snack whenever they like. This helps them develop healthier eating habits and also keeps you away from temptation. Plus, the kids will be more apt to eat quality foods at dinner if they're not full from nonstop snacking.

Drink with them. Get into the habit of drinking milk (fat-free for you and kids over age 2) when you pour it for the kids. The high-quality protein is a great appetite quencher, not to mention bone strengthener.

Busy Workers

The key to working exercise into a busy life is to give yourself lots of options and opportunities for brief periods of activity—5 minutes here and 10 minutes there—for a total of 30 minutes a day. In other words, turn to your advantage your knack for doing three things at once. Here are some strategies.

Get up 13 minutes earlier each day. Before you go to bed, lay out sneakers and exercise clothes appropriate for the weather. Use the same admirable discipline that gets you through those monster days to rise quickly and slip into your workout clothes. You should be out the front door in 3 minutes flat. Walk as briskly as you can for just 5 minutes and then turn around and head back.

Park 5 minutes farther away from the entrance. Sure, you've heard about this trick before, but you've always brushed it off, thinking that it couldn't make that much of a difference. Change your attitude. Parking farther away from your destination really can help you lose weight. Parking 10 minutes from work will add 20 minutes of exercise to your day just coming and going.

Turn your lunch break into an exercise break. No doubt you've seen other employees headed out over the lunch break with their tennis shoes on. If you like, slip into the restroom and trade your work clothes for a T-shirt. Also, keep sneakers under your desk to make changing into them easy. Pack yourself a lunch in the morning so that you can eat when you're back at work.

Delay dinner by 10 minutes each day. When you arrive home, turn around and head out the front door again. Walk at a brisk pace for 5 minutes, then turn around and return. When you can, steal an extra 5 minutes, creating a 15-minute walk.

Invest in an exercise bike. Or buy a treadmill, a rowing machine, or a stairclimber—something with which you can exercise as you read or watch television. A recumbent bike is particularly well-suited to reading and is one of the most comfortable pieces of exercise equipment. When you can't steal 10 minutes before dinner, grab 15 afterward to read the paper or a chapter of a novel or to watch the evening news, but do it on your exercise machine.

PART THREE

Stoke Your Fat-Burning System

Exercise Reality

We often say that exercise melts fat, as if fat were cool butter and exercise a warm frying pan. But that analogy isn't quite accurate. What really happens is even better.

"When you exercise, fat is metabolized in the muscles as energy," explains L. Jerome Brandon, Ph.D., associate professor of kinesiology in the department of kinesiology and health at Georgia State University in Atlanta. "There's no such thing as melting fat. You're burning fat as energy."

Yet fat doesn't go willingly into the fire. Like us, it fights for a sedentary life, which is why the pounds we accumulate are so hard to get rid of. To burn just 1 pound of fat, for example, "you're going to need to burn 3,500 calories," Dr. Brandon says.

You'd have to walk 30 miles in order to burn that much energy. "That's a lot of calories," says Dr. Brandon.

Although sustained exercise is a highly efficient way to drop the pounds, more moderate approaches also work. Consider, for example, that hypothetical 30-mile walk. You could do it all at once. Or you could spread it out, walking a mile a day for 30 days. This will ultimately burn the same pound of fat.

Done consistently, exercise will help keep fat off for the long haul, says Wayne C. Miller, Ph.D., assistant professor of kinesiology at Indiana University in Bloomington and director of the university's weight-loss clinic. "I think the critical role for exercise is in weight maintenance. Almost anything can help you lose weight, even a quack diet. People who continue exercising are the ones who maintain their weight loss."

High-Intensity Workouts

By far, the best exercise for burning blubber, experts say, is aerobic exercise. *Aerobic* means "with oxygen," and aerobic activities are those that raise your heart and breathing rates for an extended time.

"All exercise is good, but you need to elevate your pulse to 70 or 80 percent above its resting rate to burn fat effectively. Aerobic exercise does this," says Art Mollen, D.O., director of the Southwest Health Institute in Phoenix and author of *Run for Your Life* and *The Mollen Method*.

In addition to burning more fat, strenuous aerobic exercise keeps weight off by boosting metabolism—upping your RPMs, as it were. When your motor idles faster, you burn more fuel, even when you're not driving.

To begin combating corpulence with exercise, here's what experts recommend.

Do it till you're breathing hard. Aerobics is a total-body fat burner that supercharges your metabolism and ignites calories faster than normal for up to 2 hours after exercising. Some of the best aerobic activities are running, swimming, and cycling. To be most effective, these and other aerobic workouts are best done for a minimum of 30 minutes, three times a week.

Hit the Target

Aerobic exercise is the cornerstone of any long-term fat-burning plan because it does the most to fire up your metabolism. Fat starts to melt away about 20 minutes into a workout, and the higher your heart rate, the more calories you burn. Aerobic exercise also makes your charged-up metabolism ignite calories even after you've finished your workout.

To get the most benefit from any aerobic workout, however, you need to hit your "target" heart range. Here's how.

- Determine your maximum heart rate by subtracting your age from 220.
- Multiply your maximum heart rate by 0.65 to find your minimum training rate.
- Multiply your maximum heart rate by 0.8 to get your maximum training rate.

Here's how it works. Suppose you're 35 years old. Subtracting your age from 220 says your maximum heart rate is 185 beats per minute. Multiplying that by 0.65 tells you your minimum training rate is 120. Multiplying it by 0.8 says your maximum training rate is 148. Your goal, then, is to get your heart pumping between 120 and 148 beats a minute.

How do you check your heart rate while you're exercising? Feel the pulse in your wrist and count the beats for 15 seconds. Multiplying by four will give you your pulse rate.

If you're below the minimum of your target range (in the above example, that's 120 beats a minute), pick up the pace. If you're above the maximum (148 beats), slow down.

Make a long-term investment. Unless your goal is to lose weight once and then never eat again, fighting fat is an enduring commitment. In order to succeed, you have to view exercise realistically and plan your regimen accordingly. If you hate the loneliness of running, for example, don't jog. Join an aerobic dance class instead or take up squash or tennis with a friend.

Score with realistic goals. Losing weight takes long-term commitment. Trying to do it all at once will only make you frustrated and fat. Instead, define a major goal, then achieve it by reaching smaller ones.

If in the big picture you want to lose 50 pounds, shoot first for more modest goals, like losing a pound or two a week. Every day, take it a little bit further and don't backslide. You'll lose weight a lot more efficiently and, ultimately, faster than by jumping on a crash plan that's sure to fail.

Hang in for 3. You wouldn't expect that big promotion overnight, would you? So why expect more when it comes to losing weight? "I find the break-off point for exercise for most people is about 3 months," Dr. Miller says. "If you can hang in there past the third month, you've probably established some behavior that might carry on, so give yourself at least 3 months."

Get a Move On

Ask any group of people how many know they should exercise, and chances are, everyone will raise their hand. Ask the same group how many exercise regularly, and maybe only one hand will go up. Ask how many of them like to exercise, and the odds are that no one will respond positively.

The scenario is typical. Some surveys show that fewer than 1 in 10 Americans exercise as much as they should. And each year after age 40, the typical American becomes less active.

If you know that you should exercise but don't, you probably fall into one of two categories, says Catherine Brumley, certified trainer and fitness codirector at Canyon Ranch Health Resort in the Berkshires in Lenox, Massachusetts. Maybe you've never exercised and you think it's too demanding, complicated, or time-consuming. Or perhaps you have tried exercise and you didn't like it, got bored, or dropped out for some other reason.

None of those reasons is good enough to justify avoiding exercise. You can overcome every one of them.

What's more, you should. Good intentions alone don't burn calories. If you want to lose fat and keep it off, you have to exercise. Fortunately, starting an exercise program and sticking to it aren't nearly as difficult as you might imagine. Exercise need not be complicated or time-consuming. You can even learn to enjoy it.

The Fat-Fighter's Exercise Prescription

To fight fat and keep it off, you must wage a two-pronged exercise strategy, according to Maria A. Fiatarone Singh, M.D., associate professor in the School of Nutrition Science and Policy and chief of the human nutrition and exercise physiology laboratory at the Jean Mayer USDA Human Nutrition Research Center on Aging, both at Tufts University in Boston.

Strategy #1: Do some form of aerobic exercise, enough to burn off 1,600 calories a week. According to research, that's how much you need to exercise to ensure that the weight you lose will stay off. That doesn't mean you have to spend hours a day at a gym. Taking a walk every day or so can do it. If you weigh 130 pounds, for example, you'll burn 1,600 calories by walking for an hour five times a week at a 4-mile-an-hour pace.

You can burn 1,600 calories in less than 5 hours by choosing something more strenuous, such as aerobic dance or jogging. Or you can break up your activity into multiple 10- to 20-minute sessions throughout the day, such as walking for 15 minutes after breakfast, 20 minutes during your lunch break, and 15 more after work. Throw in 5 minutes in the morning and afternoon as breaks, and you've walked for an hour.

Strategy #2: Each week, on nonconsecutive days, spend 20 to 30 minutes lifting weights. (See the routine in A Crash Course in Resistance Training, page 177; it's recommended by the folks at Canyon Ranch and was designed for those who come to their spa. With fewer than 10 easy moves, you can do the routine at home or at a gym.)

Give Yourself the Aerobic Edge

The word *aerobics* was coined in 1968 by Kenneth H. Cooper, M.D. *Aerobic* means "with oxygen." So Dr. Cooper categorized exercise that makes people breathe harder, thus taking in more oxygen, as aerobic.

Aerobics caught on big-time. Today when people hear the word, they often think of doing dance moves to music. But any type of physical activity that makes you breathe harder—running, walking briskly, or swimming, for example—can be aerobic. Besides protecting against disease, aerobic exercise helps you fight fat in numerous ways.

• Aerobic exercise raises your metabolic rate during and after your workout. So you continue to burn extra calories after you exercise, says Janet Walberg-Rankin, Ph.D., associate professor of exercise science at Virginia Polytechnic Institute and State University in Blacksburg.

When researchers at the University of Vermont in Burlington compared women who exercised regularly with others who did not, they found that the first group had significantly higher metabolic rates. More than 10 hours after they'd finished exercising, the exercisers were burning calories 6 percent faster than the nonexercisers.

• You'll eat less if you exercise aerobically. When researchers measure the number of calories burned by aerobic exercisers, the results are surprising: The exercisers lose more pounds than can be accounted for by the burned calories. Why? One theory is that exercise reduces anxiety and depression, so exercisers eat less.

• You'll also eat less fat because you simply won't crave it as much. "Research indicates that exercise may enhance your preference for fruits and vegetables," explains Diane Hanson, Ph.D., a lifestyle specialist at the Pritikin Longevity Center in Malibu, California.

• You'll handle stress better, which also helps fight fat. Studies have found that physically active people handle stressful situations better than couch potatoes. Research also has shown that stress increases blood levels of a hormone called cortisol that seems to make your body store fat in your abdomen. So less stress means less pooch.

• You'll store less body fat. Aerobic exercise increases fat-burning enzymes, which break down fat and use it for energy in cells.

Ready for Liftoff

Lifting weights is one of the most important things you can do to fight fat. With weight training, you won't burn as many calories during a workout as you do with most aerobic exercises, but you will build muscle. That's significant because muscle tissue burns more calories than fat tissue does, all day long. When your body is composed of proportionally more muscle and less fat, your metabolism runs higher.

Metabolism also plays a role in fat loss during weight training. In one study, researchers found that metabolism revved up 15 percent after just 12 weeks of weight training. It's the equivalent of getting fewer calories without dieting or of eating 15 percent more just to maintain your weight.

Building muscle mass is critical to fighting fat because, after age 30, you may lose ½ pound of muscle per year even if you exercise aerobically. And, not coincidentally, you may gain about 1½ pounds of body fat per year, with much of it deposited around your middle. The less muscle you have, the lower your resting metabolic rate. So when you

A Weighty Question

You're exercising and watching what you eat, so why are you getting slimmer but *gaining* weight?

If you're lifting weights, it's no mystery, says Kristine Clark, R.D., Ph.D., director of sports nutrition at Pennsylvania State University in University Park. Weight lifting stimulates calcium absorption in your bones, so you're building a heavier skeleton. You're also building muscle, and muscle tissue weighs more than fat tissue. It's also much more compact. So your clothing size could shrink while your weight goes up or stays the same. You've changed your body composition and literally become a smaller person.

Muscle cells require more oxygen and use much more fuel than fat cells, so muscle burns more calories. The more muscle you have, the more calories you burn. For that reason, nutritionists no longer care too much about what you weigh. They're more concerned with how much body fat you have.

lose pounds of muscle over the years, calories aren't burned the way they should be, and fat accumulates. Of course, there are several ways to compensate for a sluggish metabolism. To maintain your weight after you've reached 30, you'd need to cut your weekly intake by 105 calories every year. This means that in 10 years, you'd have to shave 1,000 or more *additional* calories a week.

Barring starvation, your other option would be to add a mile a week over and above your regular walking workout every year, beginning at age 30. But by age 40, you'd have to walk an extra 10 miles per week just to maintain the same weight that you were at 21 years old.

The best option is to add about 60 minutes of resistance

training per week. That's it. You don't have to starve yourself. And while you do still need to exercise aerobically, you don't have to exercise endlessly. In other words, resistance training is the most practical, effective way to prevent the loss of muscle and maintain the metabolic rate of a 21-year-old.

Jump into Exercise and Stick with It

Chances are, if exercise has never worked for you, you've told yourself that it's because you don't have the time, you're not really motivated, or others have gotten in the way of your efforts.

Although excuses may be universal, they shouldn't thwart your exercise program. Here are some ways to overcome barriers to working out.

Give exercise a trial run. Try to stick with the effort for 1 month, suggests Brumley. The hardest part of any exercise program is getting started, she explains. In the beginning, you sometimes tend to overdo it, so your muscles may ache. Or you feel somewhat awkward. But after a month, you have more energy and better self-esteem. "If you look at exercise as 'Oh, for the rest of my life I have to do something that I hate,' you won't want to do it. But when you think of it as a trial run, exercise becomes more palatable. Usually, once people get into the habit, it becomes something they like."

Tick off each day's progress. Mark the days off the calendar with a big, thick red marker so that you can see yourself getting closer to your goal. Tell yourself, "If I still hate to exercise when this month is over, I can try something different next month." Once you've made it through 1 month, you probably won't quit, says Brumley.

Exercise your right to an option. If you feel like a klutz in an aerobic dance class, don't do aerobic dance. If jog-

Your Personal Motivation Coach

Yes, exercise helps you fight fat. But there are many other benefits. Here's additional motivation to get off the couch.

Benefit #1: Heart-smart workouts help make costly, risky medical procedures like coronary bypass operations unnecessary, by lowering levels of artery-clogging blood cholesterol.

Benefit #2: Exercise improves the way you breathe and builds muscle. That makes groceries easier to carry, jars easier to open, stairs easier to climb, and even chores easier to do.

Benefit #3: Exercise is one of the most effective ways to shake off a bad mood. Performed regularly, exercise will help keep your mood from swinging dramatically whenever stressful events occur.

Benefit #4: Exercise can help women relieve menstrual discomfort by taming surging hormones, regulating ovulation, and reducing associated discomfort such as tender breasts, bloating, and anxiety. And menopausal women who exercise moderately on a regular basis have more energy and less moodiness, anxiety, depression, sleep difficulties, night sweats, and hot flashes.

Benefit #5: Exercise strengthens bones, helping to prevent osteoporosis, a disease that makes aging bones porous and prone to breakage.

ging makes your knees hurt, don't jog. If swimming makes you dread being seen in a bathing suit, don't swim, says Brumley. Instead, pick an activity that you do enjoy or at least don't hate.

Plan for contingencies. Before making any big change, whether beginning an exercise program or giving up smoking, you need a game plan, says Elizabeth Howze, Sc.D., associate director for health promotion in the division of nutrition and physical activity at the Centers for Disease Control and Prevention. The first step in that plan is to make a list of potential deterrents and ways to get around them. Here are some questions to ask yourself.

- What will I do if it rains or snows?
- How can I balance my exercise with my family life?
- What will I do with my children while I exercise?
- What will I do during fall and winter, when it gets dark early?

"When difficulties arise, willpower alone won't help. You need a practical strategy," says Dr. Howze. "People who make changes are more successful if they first plan for how they are going to deal with difficulties."

Start with an activity that appeals to you. If you're intimidated by exercise, try something that you already know how to do. For many, that means walking. But think about all the aerobic activities you have tried. Ask yourself which of those was comfortable.

Avoid post-traumatic gym syndrome. If you're like many people, you may have bad memories of a dreaded day in gym class when you were forced to run a mile in under 10 minutes or you were the last one picked for softball. If you know from experience that a particular exercise isn't for you—if running seemed like torture or if team sports embarrassed you—cross it off your list of options.

Be patient. If your list of not-to-do exercises outnumbers your list of to-do activities, don't give up hope. Experts say that in their experience, most people can find at least one activity they enjoy. Although you may need to experiment, you'll find something you like.

Turn to your chores for exercise. If you don't like the idea of formal exercise sessions, make daily activities your exercise, says Dr. Howze. Keep track of the amount of time you spend walking up the stairs, washing your car, or vacuuming—anything active that you do during the day. Then make sure that you spend a total of at least 30 minutes a day on these activities, which can be just as effective as walking, swimming, or other aerobic activity, says Dr. Howze.

Challenge yourself. Once you select an activity, vary it somehow to make it more interesting. If you like to walk, for instance, make it a little harder by walking up a big hill. Or walk faster for a block. And try to do a more difficult activity once a week, like stairclimbing or cross-country skiing.

Find the time. First, take stock of how you now spend your time. For about a week, keep a record of your time, much as you would enter expenditures in your checkbook, says Virginia Bass, a time-management consultant and owner of By Design, a personal and professional development company in Exton, Pennsylvania. Then review your time log. Chances are, you can nip and tuck parts of each day to free up bits of time. Instead of talking to a neighbor on the phone, maybe you could take a walk around the neighborhood together. Instead of satisfying your addiction to CNN from the easy chair, you could soak up the news while you pedal a stationary bike.

Start with as much time as you can spare. Exercise doesn't have to be an all-or-nothing venture. "As little as 10 minutes a day helps," says Susan W. Butterworth, Ph.D., director of wellness services for the occupational-health program at Oregon Health Sciences University in Portland. Once exercise becomes a habit, chances are that you'll find more time to do it.

Designate a time slot for exercise. Once exercise is on your to-do list, decide when to do it. Otherwise, you won't always get to it.

Early birds who work out in the mornings believe that they are much more likely to stick to their programs than people who leave exercise until later, when unexpected demands can knock the best intentions off-balance. Others find that working out at noon is best because they don't have to find a sitter for the kids. Some people prefer a walk, followed by a bath, as a nightcap. So the "right" time to exercise is whatever time works for you.

Block out the time. Write your exercise appointment on your calendar or in your date book. "You don't have to tell your secretary or business associates what the appointment is for. It's just an appointment," says Dr. Butterworth. Treat it the same way you would a business appointment or other obligation, she says.

Strategize with your family. Explain that exercise is important to you and ask your family to help you find ways to fit it in.

Make exercise a family outing. You can have your 5-year-old ride his bike alongside you as you jog. Or you can enroll him in a gym activity, such as a karate class, while you take aerobics, says Dr. Butterworth. You might also try to schedule family fitness hours, with the entire family doing something active like cycling, walking at the zoo, or tossing a Frisbee.

The Fast Track
to Weight Loss

There's no easy way to make the pounds disappear. What took you 20 years to put on won't come off overnight. Still, it is possible to shed pounds without waiting years for results.

Being realistic is key. So is advance planning. If you're going to lose weight for your high school class reunion, for instance, you'll want to begin before it's 2 months away. And even before you begin lining up specific weight-loss strategies, here's what experts recommend.

Back to Basics

Yes, it would be fun to lose weight, buy smashing new duds, and arrive at the reunion in a blue Mercedes—all in the same 2 weeks. But it's not going to happen.

The point is not to be discouraged but to plan ahead. "A person may lose somewhere between 3 and 5 pounds of fat reasonably and safely in a month's time," says L. Jerome Brandon, Ph.D., associate professor of kinesiology in the department of kinesiology and health at Georgia

State University in Atlanta. Use that as a working number. If you hope to shed 20 pounds for the reunion in June, get serious sometime in January about losing weight. Here are other doctor-approved strategies.

Make goals you can control. It's good to strive for long-range targets, but don't make promises to yourself that you can't keep. When you're trying to lose weight, nothing energizes like success or brings you down faster than failure.

"My advice is to set goals that you are completely in charge of," says Joan Price, a fitness instructor and owner of Unconventional Moves, a fitness consulting service in Sebastopol, California. "For example, that you will exercise five times a week as long as you're able is a goal that you're in charge of. That you will lose 20 pounds by your reunion is not, since you can't control how fast you lose weight."

Take affirmative action. One way to keep laserlike focus on your goal to practice affirmations, positive statements you memorize and repeat, like a mantra. Doing this imprints your goal into your psyche, making you more likely to achieve your objective.

Make your affirmations short and specific, like "I will walk 5 days a week for the next 5 weeks." Write your goal on paper and post it somewhere you'll see it every day, like on the bathroom mirror. Spend a few minutes each day repeating your goal to yourself. Say it slowly, deliberately, and with conviction.

"As you repeat affirmations, try to imagine each one is—or can be—true. Actually see yourself changing," says Dennis T. Jaffe, Ph.D., a consultant at HeartWork in San Francisco and coauthor of *Self-Renewal* and *Rekindling Commitment.*

Be sane. People who are overambitious may experience quick rewards, but they're almost guaranteed to have long-term setbacks as well. As a rule, experts say, don't try to lose more than 5 pounds a month. You'll just become weak, or worse. "When you lose body weight too quickly, you're endangering your health," warns Dr. Brandon.

Keep It Fun

When you're trying to lose weight fast, don't get bogged down with a laundry list of activities that you loathe. Time is short, so stick with things you enjoy and know you'll do.

"Especially for the short term, people have to do the type of exercises they're comfortable with," says Roger G. Sargent, Ph.D., professor of public health and nutrition at the University of South Carolina School of Public Health in Columbia. "For some people, this will be biking. For others, it will be running. You have to find something you're comfortable with in order to stick with it." And then follow this advice.

Duplicate your efforts. It takes discipline, but exercising twice a day enhances the probability that you'll burn fat fast.

"We also know that if you have limited time periods, two or three segments of exercise equal the benefit of a single bout of equal time. If I were serious about losing weight in the short term, I'd do my exercises twice a day," Dr. Sargent says. "Doubling your dose of exercise gives you a great metabolic kick. You'll put an enormous burden on your metabolism and get a great return."

Bring on the power. Serious weight loss requires serious effort, like combining aerobic exercise with strength training, says Dr. Sargent. Aerobic exercises such as running, cycling, and walking mobilize fat throughout your body, while weight lifting builds lean muscle mass in those body parts you work hardest. More muscle tissue means faster metabolism, which enables you to burn more calories even when you're not exercising.

Always be prepared. Promising yourself you'll never miss a workout is like saying you'll never be sick. Keeping your exercise togs in the trunk, however, makes it easier to work out when the urge strikes. This is particularly helpful when you're trying to lose weight fast and every workout counts.

Maximize opportunity. Exercise doesn't happen only on the track or in the gym. Every day, there are dozens of little opportunities—going shopping, walking to your car, or just going from the basement to the fourth floor—that help us burn a little more flab, says Kelly Brownell, Ph.D., professor of psychology and a weight-loss expert at Yale University.

For starters, lose the remote control and actually get up to change channels. It's not a marathon, but it helps. So does getting out of the car and opening the garage door by hand, walking the shopping malls instead of ordering by mail, taking stairs instead of elevators, walking at lunch instead of having an hour-long meal. All these small efforts add up to decent workouts, and workouts subtract pounds.

Eat smart. You can exercise 5 days a week, but if you're not alert to what goes into your mouth, you're going to lose the battle, says Dr. Brownell. Consider this: One ¼-pound cheeseburger, a small order of fries, and a shake has more than 1,000 calories, about the same number you'd burn during a 10-mile run or a 3-hour game of tennis.

You don't have to be fanatical about dieting to lose weight, says Dr. Sargent. In fact, you don't need to diet at all. Just cut back on fatty foods—things like burgers, fries, and rich desserts—and eat more of the foods you know are good for you, like potatoes, beans, fruits, vegetables, and bread.

A Crash Course
in Resistance Training

When combined with aerobic exercise, weight training effectively provides the one-two knockout punch in the slugfest against fat. While aerobic exercise helps you to burn off calories, weight training helps to build toned muscle and sculpt your body. A pound of muscle is smaller, firmer, and shapelier than a pound of fat. So as you replace fat with muscle, your body will take on a firmer shape.

"Large muscle mass helps burn calories too," says Miriam Nelson, Ph.D., research scientist at the exercise physiology research center at the Jean Mayer USDA Human Nutrition Research Center on Aging at Tufts University in Boston. That's because muscle requires more oxygen and more calories to sustain itself than fat does. And strength training is more effective than aerobic exercise at building and maintaining muscle. So you burn more calories, all day long, all week long.

Lifting Lessons

What could be easier than lifting weights? Up, down, up, down, up, down. But there are some general guidelines to follow to get the most benefits.

Three times spells success. You can get away with lifting only twice a week, according to Catherine Brumley, certified trainer and fitness codirector at Canyon Ranch Health Resort in the Berkshires in Lenox, Massachusetts. But you'll get leaner faster if you lift 3 days a week.

Take every other day off. Rest for at least 1 day between workouts, says Brumley. A day or two off will give your muscles a chance to recuperate.

Warm up. Five to 10 minutes of brisk walking ought to grease your joints and tendons so that movements are easier to do and you don't injure anything when you start your weight workout, according to Brumley. Follow the warmup with some limbering range-of-motion movements, as explained below.

Make a dry run. To ready your muscles, quickly go through the motion of the exercise 5 to 10 times without weight before actually lifting the weight, says Brumley.

Take breaks. After each exercise, be sure to rest for up to 2 minutes before moving on to the next exercise. Rest breaks give your muscles a chance to recuperate and prepare for further effort. When you first begin to work out, you may need to rest for the full 2 minutes before you feel able to do the next exercise. As time passes, however, you will probably be able to shorten your rest time, says Molly Foley, an exercise physiologist and director of ReQuest Physical Therapy in Gainesville, Florida.

Work in sets. You want to lift the weight 8 to 12 times (called repetitions). After each set of repetitions, rest for 1 to 2 minutes to let your muscle recover, then do a second set of the same exercise. As an alternative, to save time, you can work a different muscle or opposing muscle groups between sets instead of resting. You can alternate between arm and leg exercises, for instance: First, curl a weight 10 times to work your biceps; then do 10 squats to work your legs while you allow the biceps muscles in your upper arms to rest; then work your biceps again. Or for variety, says Brumley, you can add a circuit workout to your weight-training routine. In this type of workout, you might lift a weight 10 times, jog in place for 2 to 3 minutes, lift the weight again, jog again, and then move on to your next exercise.

Start light. Most people overestimate the amount of weight they can lift, says Karen Rucker, M.D., chair of the department of physical medicine and rehabilitation at Virginia Commonwealth University School of Medicine in Richmond. "They think 10 pounds is nothing, yet they need two hands to lift a 2-liter seltzer bottle (about 4 pounds)," says Dr. Rucker. To find out which weights to begin with, consider what you lift in a day. A grocery bag with two cans of soup, two oranges, one grapefruit, a half-gallon of milk, and a head of broccoli, for example, weighs about 10 pounds. Can you lift that 12 times in a row? If that's too much weight, see how the seltzer bottle feels.

"We start out very slowly for the first 2 to 3 weeks, at about 50 percent of the weight people can lift. This is to prevent injury. If the training isn't enjoyable, you may not continue," says Margarita Smith Treuth, Ph.D., fellow at Baylor College of Medicine in Houston.

Push the limit. For true strength gains, you want to work your muscles to failure—the point at which your muscle is so tuckered out that it can't lift the weight one more time—during each set. Working a muscle to exhaustion helps to make it stronger, says Brumley.

Breathe. Exhale while you lift the weight—during exertion—and inhale as you lower it, says Nancy C. Karabaic, a certified personal trainer in Silver Spring, Maryland.

Take a minute. That's how long it takes a muscle to get stronger: 1 minute. Take 2 whole seconds to lift the weight, exhaling while you are lifting. Then take 4 seconds to lower the weight. This doesn't mean just counting to four; it means 4 seconds (you know, one one-thousand, two one-thousand). The whole exercise took 6 seconds, times 10 repetitions. You have just built your biceps (or whatever muscle you're working on).

Follow the rule of 12. "Resistance training for muscle strength and size should always be done with a weight that you can lift only 8 to 12 times before fatiguing," says Maria A. Fiatarone Singh, M.D., associate professor in the School of Nutrition Science and Policy and chief of the human nutrition and exercise physiology laboratory at the Jean Mayer USDA Human Nutrition Research Center on Aging, both at Tufts University in Boston. The key is to make your muscles tired, because after being completely fatigued, a muscle will recharge itself and bounce back even stronger. If you can lift your current amount of weight 12 times but there's no way you could go for number 13, you know that you're using the correct weight. When you can do 12 repetitions with strength to spare, it's time to increase the weight.

Stretch after your workout. In the course of lifting weights, muscles contract and shorten, making them less flexible. So you'll want to stretch after lifting, while your muscles are still warm, to restore muscle length and keep them flexible. Hold each stretch for 20 to 30 seconds, says Brumley.

Listen to your body. Various lifestyle factors, such as how much sleep you've had or lost, when you ate your last meal, and how much stress you're under, can change how much weight you can lift in a day. So listen to your body and ease up if you don't feel up to your usual workload some days.

Measure success by weight lifted, not by weight lost. Healthy changes in the amount of fat and muscle in your

Toning Anytime, Anywhere

You don't have to have dumbbells and a weight bench to work your muscles. In fact, you can help strengthen and tone your muscles during many of your day-to-day activities. Here are some ideas from fitness experts.

Be your own squeeze. When driving, standing in line, or sitting in a waiting room, squeeze your buttocks, thighs, and abdominals to give your muscles a workout, says Mia Finnegan, a fitness trainer and owner of Tru Fitness, an exercise service in Pasadena, California.

Give yourself a raise. While washing dishes or brushing your teeth, do toe raises to work your calves, says Teresa Flunker, an exercise physiologist in Gainesville, Florida.

Squat, don't bend. Instead of bending over to do chores, do a squat to work your leg and butt muscles. Do the same when picking things up from the floor, says Flunker.

Do television waist whittlers. While watching TV or doing any other activity that involves sitting, you can still work the muscles along your waist, says Peggy Norwood, former director of the fitness program at Duke University and president of Avalon Fitness, both in Durham, North Carolina. Place one hand on your opposite knee and lift that leg 6 to 8 inches off the floor. Flex your stomach muscles as you gently apply counter-pressure to the top of your knee with your hand, allowing your elbow to bend slightly.

body may not show up on the scale, but they'll certainly show up on the weight stacks in the gym. Write down the weights you use when you start. One pound? Two? Measure that against what you are lifting even as little as 16 weeks later. If that doesn't float your boat as a way to measure success, try your waistband. Even when the workout benefits don't show up on the scale, they'll be evident in the fit of your clothing.

Perfect Your Technique

When you lift, proper form is as important as frequency. Heed these tips.

Give yourself enough room. People who begin to lift weights often don't give themselves enough "elbow room," says Karabaic. They tend to keep their arms at their sides and their legs close together. To train properly, she says, you need to spread out and take up as much room as you need to be comfortable.

Pay particular attention when you're doing squats, says Karabaic. To do a squat correctly, you have to stick your butt out, which at first makes some people feel self-conscious, she says.

Visualize the exercise. To lift weights correctly, you need to feel your muscles move. Yet some people who are overweight or uncomfortable with their bodies for any reason tend to be out of touch with what it takes to move their bodies, says Kathy Mangan, a certified personal trainer and weight-loss counselor in Missoula, Montana. So at first, weight lifting may feel foreign. Visualization can help overcome that awkwardness and help you lift correctly, says Mangan. Before you actually start the strength-training exercises described on the following pages, picture yourself doing the motions. In particular, think about which parts of your body you will use to do the motions correctly and how that might feel.

Don't lock your joints. When doing any exercise, don't lock your elbows or knees, as some people are inclined to do at the beginning or end of a repetition. If you do, you'll end up putting weight on the joint instead of the muscle, possibly causing elbow or knee pain, says Karabaic.

Use good posture. Good posture will help protect your joints and spine from strain, says Tereasa Flunker, an exercise physiologist in Gainesville, Florida. Before each movement, check to make sure that you have good posture. Whether you are standing up or lying on your back on a bench, plant your feet on the ground or bench about shoulder-width apart. Bend your knees slightly and let your arms relax at your sides. Lift your breastbone by pulling your shoulders back and down. Roll your pelvis so that your lower back is straight instead of curved inward.

Smart Equipment Choices

You don't have to join a large gym with dozens of exercise machines to tone up. A few simple items will suffice. Here's what to look for.

Buy varying sets of weights. Because some muscles will be stronger than others, you'll need more than one pair of dumbbells. Buy sets of 3-, 5-, and 10-pound dumbbells. Later, as you become stronger, you'll probably need heavier ones, but most beginners don't need anything heavier than 10 pounds, says Flunker. You can save money on dumbbells by going to a secondhand sporting goods store such as Play It Again Sports, scouting garage sales, or offering to buy lighter weights from bodybuilders who've moved on to heavier ones, says Flunker.

Go for comfort. Unlike purchasing a treadmill, stairclimber, or other exercise machine, buying dumbbells doesn't require a lot of research or comparison shopping. Dumbbells haven't evolved much since the day of their invention. Your main objective is to find dumbbells that are comfortable to hold, says Mangan. They vary in length and width; you'll probably feel more comfortable with shorter ones. The longer the dumbbell, the more unwieldy it is, she says.

You also want a comfortable bench. Since some are wider than others, lie on the bench at the store to make sure that it is wide enough to support your body, says Mangan. You don't want your shoulders or sides hanging over the edges, making you feel as if you might fall off. Also, some benches are taller than others. Make sure that your feet can comfortably touch the floor when you are lying down, she says.

Slip on the gloves. You can get through your routine without them, but you'll feel more comfortable with a pair of weight-lifting gloves. They help you grip the weight securely and prevent calluses.

Quick-and-Easy Weight Lifting

You want to train all of your major muscle groups to get the best benefits. That means your arms, legs, abdomen, back, and rear end. Here's a short total-body weight-lifting routine designed by the fitness professionals at Canyon Ranch.

Dumbbell Bench Press

Muscles toned: chest (pectoralis major), fronts of shoulders (anterior deltoids), and backs of upper arms (triceps)

What to do: Lie on your back on a bench with your feet flat on the floor. Your buttocks, upper back, and head should stay in contact with the bench during the exercise. Hold a dumbbell in each hand and lift them so that they are directly above your shoulders. Your elbows should be straight but not locked and the ends of the dumbbells should touch each other.

Slowly lower the dumbbells by bending your elbows and bringing your arms down to the sides. Keep the dumbbells perpendicular to your torso until they are even with your chest. Your elbows should be bent at 90-degree angles. You should feel a stretch in your chest. Then press the dumbbells upward and together to return to the starting position, and repeat.

Dumbbell Row

Muscles toned: upper back (latissimus dorsi), back of shoulder (posterior deltoid), and front of upper and lower arm (elbow flexor)

What to do: Stand sideways next to a bench. To support your lower back, place one hand—with your elbow extended but not locked—and the corresponding knee on the bench. Your hand should be directly under your shoulder, and your standing leg should be slightly bent and under your hip. Keep your back straight and your shoulders parallel to the floor during the exercise. In your free hand, hold a dumbbell with your palm facing your body and your arm extended directly below your shoulder.

Lift your elbow toward the ceiling, keeping it close to your body, and raise the dumbbell until it is even with your chest, keeping your torso as stationary as possible. Your elbow will be above your back. Then slowly lower the dumbbell to the starting position, and repeat. Complete all repetitions with one arm before switching to the other arm.

Squat

Muscles toned: buttocks (gluteus maximus), fronts of thighs (quadriceps), and backs of thighs (hamstrings)

What to do: Stand with your feet slightly more than shoulder-width apart and your toes pointed straight forward or slightly out. If you are using weights for more resistance, hold your arms straight down at your sides throughout the exercise.

With your back flat, your chest up, and your eyes focused straight ahead, lower your body into a squat, as if you were sitting down in a chair, until your knees are bent at 90-degree angles. Your knees should be directly above (never beyond) your toes. Keep your back straight and your heels on the floor. Keep your weight balanced back toward your heels to prevent yourself from leaning too far forward. Rise from the squat by forcing your hips in line. Extend your hips fully at the top and squeeze your buttocks muscles before beginning the next repetition.

Overhead Press

Muscles toned: shoulders (deltoids), backs of upper arms (triceps), and lower neck and upper middle back (trapezius)

What to do: Sit sideways on a bench with your feet flat on the floor and a dumbbell in each hand. Your elbows should be bent and your palms facing forward at shoulder level, with the dumbbells slightly more than shoulder-width apart.

While keeping your back flat, press the dumbbells up and extend your arms overhead until the ends of the dumbbells meet. Lower the dumbbells and repeat.

Biceps Curl

Muscles toned: fronts of upper arms (biceps)

What to do: Stand with your back to a wall, with your feet about a foot from the wall and your knees slightly bent. Press your lower and upper back flat against the wall. With your palms facing out, hold the dumbbells with the ends touching at about mid thigh.

Bend your elbows, keeping them pressed against your sides, as you lift the dumbbells up toward your shoulders. Do not arch your back in order to provide extra momentum for your lift. Slowly lower the dumbbells to the starting position and repeat.

Back Extension

Muscles toned: lower back (spinal erectors), buttocks (gluteus maximus), and backs of thighs (hamstrings)

What to do: Lie facedown on the floor with your elbows bent to the sides and your hands palms down under your forehead. (*Caution:* Those with disk problems or current back spasms should consider an alternative exercise.)

Lift your head, chest, arms, legs, and feet simultaneously, keeping just the middle of your body in contact with the floor. Lift only as far as you can without discomfort. Be sure to keep your head and neck aligned while you stare at the floor. Keep your legs straight. Hold the position for 2 to 5 seconds, then slowly lower yourself back to the floor. Touch the floor lightly, but don't rest before doing the next repetition.

Abdominal Crunch

Muscles toned: abdominals (rectus abdominis)

What to do: Lie on the floor with your legs bent at an angle that allows you to keep your feet flat and your lower back pressed against the floor. Place your fingers behind your head for support, with your elbows back.

Use your abdominal muscles to raise your buttocks (no more than 2 inches) and lift your shoulders, keeping your lower back pressed to the floor. Be sure not to use your fingers to jerk your head off the floor. Hold for a count of five, then slowly lower your shoulders and buttocks to the floor. Start your next crunch immediately; don't take any time to rest. If you have difficulty raising your shoulders and buttocks at the same time, try raising your shoulders first and then raise your buttocks so that both are up at the same time.

If you have lower-back pain, do the exercise with your legs resting on a bench, being sure to keep your lower back pressed to the floor.

For a more advanced workout, hold your legs up with your knees and hip joints bent at 90-degree angles. Then curl your upper and lower body together, trying to touch your elbows to your knees.

Get the Aerobic Edge

Sweat. Complicated calisthenics performed to loud music. Taut butts and perky ponytails.

If that's what you think of when you think "aerobics," think again. You can work aerobics into your exercise program without even setting foot in an aerobics class.

"Many people hate to exercise aerobically because they define it too narrowly," says Catherine Brumley, certified trainer and fitness codirector at Canyon Ranch Health Resort in the Berkshires in Lenox, Massachusetts. "They think aerobic exercise means going to an aerobics class, which makes them feel uncoordinated. Or they think aerobic exercise means being in a pool, and they don't like to wear a swimsuit. Or they feel uncomfortable in a gym environment. When they realize there are other options, however, most find an aerobic exercise they enjoy."

Even doing chores and playing with your kids or grandkids could count, as long as you're moving your body with a purpose and not sitting on your rear end. The only "rule" is that you spend enough time exercising to burn at least 1,600 calories a week, according to researchers at William

Beaumont Hospital in Birmingham, Michigan. That's the equivalent of walking for an hour at a 4-mile-per-hour pace, 5 days a week.

Walk Off the Weight

You've been walking since you were a baby, so you may think you know all the basics. But there are different ways to walk, and some give you a better aerobic workout.

Heel-to-toe walking, for instance, involves the whole body in one great gliding, heart-pumping, joint-flexing, muscle-working, calorie-burning motion. Because it protects the knees, this kind of walking is safe for people over age 40 or those who have never exercised, says Brumley.

All you need to do is coordinate your arms, hips, and feet while you maintain proper posture. Here's each step broken down.

Assume the correct posture. Stand tall, with your chin up and your weight slightly forward on the balls of your feet. Lean just slightly forward from the ankles without bending at the waist. Imagine that your body is a board and it's starting to tip forward, all in one plane. Avoid a swayback by tucking in your buttocks and your stomach, but don't strain. Keep your shoulders relaxed. This lean allows gravity to help you move forward. (You can check your posture by standing in front of a mirror and getting into position just before a walk.)

Start walking. Try to point your feet straight ahead. Make gentle corrections if you notice your feet pointing out or in. Land on your heel with your toes and forefoot raised at about a 25- to 30-degree angle off the ground. (Landing on your heel this way helps straighten your knee, which diverts impact from your knee joint.) Allow yourself to roll forward on your foot, pressing down on the outside portion of the bottom of your foot so that you feel continuous contact with the ground. Push off with your toes.

Practice walking barefoot. At first, just walk around the house barefoot to get the feel of it. You'll notice a distinct push forward when you use this rolling motion, in contrast to your normal, more flat-footed stride. Go slowly, and you'll also realize just how strong your toes are and how much motion you can get out of your whole foot. You'll also notice greater use of your buttock muscles than in regular walking.

Use your hips properly. Hips that waddle side to side are a result of faulty technique. When you heel-to-toe walk with proper form, you look powerful and graceful, not anything like a duck.

To correct your technique, stand in front of a mirror and try this exercise suggested by Elaine Ward, walking coach, author of several fitness- and competitive-walking books, and managing director of the North American Racewalking Federation. Walk in place by moving your knees forward and back. Stand tall and let your arms swing naturally at your sides. Next, let your hips swing forward and back with your legs. You'll feel a twisting motion at your waist. If it's hard to get your hips moving, pretend you're holding on to a towel and drying off your behind. Notice that the movement of your arms helps your hips move forward and back even farther. When you are walking, this hip movement allows you to keep your back foot on the ground a bit longer, extending your stride behind you and giving power to your push off.

Move your arms. Arm movement complements leg and hip movement and turns walking into a total-body workout. When you walk using your arms properly, you'll feel a sense of rhythm and coordination, plus extra power. Your shoulder joints stay flexible too. Bend your arms to at least a right angle, but a little more is better, according to some coaches. Let them swing like pendulums from your relaxed shoulders.

Hold your hands cupped in loosely clenched fists as you swing your arms forward and back, forward and back.

Don't hunch up. Your hands should swing no higher in front than the midline of your chest, and they should swing straight ahead, not on the diagonal. As you swing back, your hands should go back as far as an imaginary back pocket, but no farther. Your elbows should stay close to your body. (Check your arm swing by walking in front of a mirror.)

Pointers for Beginners

If you're out of shape, don't expect to walk for an hour five times a week. If you do too much too soon, you'll hurt. Start with what feels comfortable, maybe walking 10 minutes a day.

"Kind of underdo it each time, so you don't hurt or exhaust yourself. Don't create a reason to stop doing it," says Suki Munsell, Ph.D., director of the Dynamic Health and Fitness Institute in Corte Madera, California. First, focus on frequency: Work up to five times a week. Then work on duration: Extend the time you spend walking each day. Last, increase intensity: Speed up your pace or take on steep hills. Follow these guidelines.

Begin by taking several short walks in the course of a day. If it seems like there's no good time to walk, consider the prime-time opportunities: before or after a meal, after a long meeting, at the end of the workday, or a couple of hours after dinner.

Increase by 10 percent a week. If you started by walking for 10 minutes a day for the first week, walk for 11 minutes a day the following week, says Dr. Munsell. Gradual increases should allow you to eventually work up to at least a ½ hour, four to six times a week.

Talk to yourself. Walk at a slow enough pace that you can talk about what happened on your favorite TV show last night but not so slowly that you can hum the show's theme song.

Hold your head high. Keeping your head aligned with your shoulders, not tilted forward or arched back, will help your neck support your head, says Dr. Munsell. If you lead with your chin, you'll probably end up with neck pain.

Don't lead with your hips. Some people walk with their hips thrust forward, as if someone had just yanked their upper bodies backward. Walking that way strains the lower back, says Dr. Munsell, so try to keep your hips aligned with your shoulders.

Mix it up. To stay motivated and avoid overuse injuries, change terrain. Opt for areas where the ground offers a variety of surfaces, or switch routes.

Other Aerobic Options

If you don't like to walk, you can choose from a wide variety of other aerobic exercises. You want to find a couple of kinds of aerobic exercise that are easy and enjoyable and that you're likely to do today, next week, next month, next year, and the rest of your life.

First and foremost, find something you enjoy. But think about other criteria too. Can you afford the equipment or fees? Is it convenient? Is it comfortable? Here's what top exercise and weight-loss experts have to say about a few of the more common types of aerobic exercises.

Aerobic Dance

Pros: At home, you can do aerobics at any time of the day by popping a videotape into the VCR. If you go to a gym, spending time with others who want to be healthy and firm can help keep you motivated. You get great calorie burn.

Cons: You have to keep up with the instructor. High-impact classes can be hard on the joints.

Cross-Country Skiing

Pros: It's easy on your joints and works your upper and lower body for increased calorie burn. "Cross-country skiing rates highest in lab tests for burning the most calories per minute because you're using your legs, your upper body, and even your torso," says Wayne Westcott, Ph.D., of Quincy, Massachusetts, national strength-training consultant for the YMCA. Cross-country skiing scorches up to 660 calories per hour. (Downhill is no slouch, either, burning about 570 calories per hour.)

Cons: Skiing on an indoor machine requires coordination. Skiing outdoors requires skis, boots, and poles, adequate amounts of snow, and access to suitable terrain.

Cycling

Pros: You get high calorie burn with little pressure on your joints. Cycling also has a high convenience level. You can ride outdoors or indoors. You can ride with others. You can even cycle to work. Gear tips: Don't neglect the headgear; always wear a helmet. Don cycling gloves to protect your hands if you take a spill, to absorb sweat, to dampen vibration, and to give you a better grip on the handlebar. Wear stiff-soled biking shoes designed to grip the pedal, give you more power, and help prevent your feet from flying off.

Cons: People with back pain should consider recumbent stationary bicycles, which allow you to lean back while you pedal.

Dancing

Pros: There's little or no boredom here. Any dance style—square dancing, rock and roll, disco, belly dancing, or salsa, for instance—counts. There's minimal training needed. You can't go wrong, calorie-wise, even if your dance form leaves a little to be desired. And dancing costs next to nothing: Pop in your favorite compact disc and do it in your living room.

Cons: Almost none, unless you are rhythm-impaired.

Golfing

Pros: Golf is great exercise. You'll walk about 2 miles playing the average 9-hole course. An 18-holer will take you 4 miles. One study found that golfers who played three times a week showed dramatic improvement in their cholesterol levels. *Note:* You might think that a round of golf is about as stressful as raising a Tom Collins. But lack of flexibility is a leading cause of back injury on the PGA Tour, says Lewis A. Yocum, M.D., assistant medical director of the PGA Tour and PGA Senior Tour. To prevent injuries, get in the habit of loosening up and stretching before you hit the first tee. Stretch your upper body for several minutes, including your arms, shoulders, chest, neck, and back. Finish up by stretching your calves, your hamstrings, and the rest of your lower body.

Cons: Climbing in and out of a golf cart between swings doesn't do much for your cardiovascular system. Make sure you walk the course and carry your own golf bag.

Jogging

Pros: It incinerates calories. "Jogging burns fat, keeps your heart healthy, and can be done without a lot of preparation or trouble," says Art Mollen, D.O., director of the Southwest Health Institute in Phoenix and author of *Run for Your Life* and *The Mollen Method.*

For best results, says Budd Coates, a four-time Olympic Marathon Trials qualifier and consultant to *Runner's World* magazine, break in slowly. For the first week, just walk, he advises. Walk about 20 minutes for 4 days in a row. On days 5 through 8, increase the time to 30 minutes. As your legs (and lungs) start feeling stronger, do about 2 minutes of running followed by 4 minutes of walking. Again, do this for about a week, 30 minutes each time. After that, you may feel comfortable going into a full run for 30 minutes without stopping. But don't be discouraged if you continue to walk and run. Every step is burning weight and helping you get into shape. The running will follow.

Cons: Jogging is tough on the ankles, knees, and hips.

Martial Arts

Pros: They're superb for increasing strength, building muscle, and burning fat. They can be very aerobic, depending on the style you practice, says Richard Carrera, Ph.D., psychologist at the University of Miami. There's a martial art form for anyone, no matter what level of fitness you're at. (In addition to the more macho forms, there are "soft" arts such as tai chi chuan, which emphasizes coordination, relaxation, and suppleness.) And virtually any martial art, done vigorously, will help get your heart rate up and keep your weight down.

Cons: You have to enroll in a class. And choosing the wrong instructor or school might turn you off to what could otherwise be a lifetime avocation.

Rowing

Pros: Rowing works the upper and lower body for increased calorie burn without overstressing your joints. It's an efficient fat burner that ranks with cross-country skiing as one of the best aerobic exercises you can do, says rowing expert Fredrick C. Hagerman, Ph.D., biological sciences professor at Ohio University in Athens. "If you look at the energy cost for any given level of exercise, rowing is probably one of the highest calorie burners you can find." Once you get moving, you can burn up to 1,200 calories an hour.

Cons: You need to either buy a rowing machine, join a gym that has rowing equipment, or find a boat.

Stair climbing

Pros: It works primary trouble spots—the butt, thighs, and hips. It's easy on the joints.

Cons: It's easy to cheat by leaning on the console or gripping the handrails too tightly, either of which lowers your calorie burn.

Swimming

Pros: Swimming is kind to your joints. The water resistance can also build muscle, but not as well as during a water aerobics class.

Cons: Unlike out-of-water exercises that increase your body's inner temperature and squelch your appetite, swimming in cold water may actually increase your craving for calories to keep your body warm. (If possible, select a pool heated to about 82°F.) Of course, you need to know how to swim.

Water aerobics

Pros: The gentle support of the water nearly guarantees against injury and discomfort while helping to make your body more flexible. Water resistance helps build muscle strength while you burn calories.

Cons: You need to attend a class or have a pool in your backyard. You have to wear a swimsuit in front of other people.

Mini-Aerobics Add Up

You don't have to burn all of your calories in one long aerobic burst. You can slowly but consistently add them up throughout the day by doing things like taking the stairs or walking from the parking lot. You want to accumulate a ½ hour or more of such activities a day, says Maria A. Fiatarone Singh, M.D., associate professor in the School of

Nutrition Science and Policy and chief of the human nutrition and exercise physiology laboratory at the Jean Mayer USDA Human Nutrition Research Center on Aging, both at Tufts University in Boston.

This approach works best for people who hate to exercise. "It's sort of like putting small amounts of money in the bank. You get in 10 minutes here, 5 minutes there, and 10 minutes another time. Your time adds up," says Elizabeth Howze, Sc.D., associate director for health promotion in the division of nutrition and physical activity at the Centers for Disease Control and Prevention (CDC).

Here are some examples of how small bursts of aerobic activity add up.

Take up climbing. Whenever you have the chance, climb the stairs instead of getting in the elevator. You burn 10 times more calories climbing stairs than you do standing still. If this means that you need to allow yourself a few more minutes to get to your office or to make your way through an airport, so be it, even if you have to leave earlier for your destination.

Relay the groceries. Carry your grocery bags into the house one at a time, says Kathy Mangan, a certified personal trainer and weight-loss counselor in Missoula, Montana.

Boycott the car wash. Don't take your car to a drive-through car wash. Instead, get out the hose and the soap and do it yourself, says Mangan.

Kid around. Rather than pop in a video to keep your children or grandchildren entertained, play actively with them. Play catch, jump rope, climb on the monkey bars, push them on swings, or run footraces, suggests Vicki Pierson, a personal trainer and weight-management consultant in Chattanooga, Tennessee.

Make dancing dates. Go once or twice a month to a dance club, says Pierson. Or take dance lessons.

Watch Out for Faux Aerobics

You may think that many activities are aerobic when they're not, says Barbara Ainsworth, Ph.D., associate professor of epidemiology and biostatistics and of exercise science at the University of South Carolina School of Public Health in Columbia. Here are some that may or may not be aerobic, depending on how you go about doing them.

Doing the laundry. Modern conveniences have made washing clothes a no-breather. You can, however, work in a little exercise by hanging your clothes on the line instead of tossing them in the dryer.

Cutting the lawn. With a riding mower? Get real. To get better exercise, use a push mower.

Putting in a hard day at the office. Unless you are painting the office or building it, your desk job probably isn't strenuous. Try walking letters down to the mailroom, taking the stairs instead of the elevator, and hand-delivering documents to coworkers to improve the aerobic state of your job.

Give up sunbathing. While at the beach, stay active by swimming, wave surfing, renting a rowboat or paddleboat, or playing volleyball or paddleball, says Pierson.

Get back to basics. If you have a riding mower, switch to a push mower. If you have a power push mower, switch to a manual, says Pierson.

Be Bob Vila or Martha Stewart. Whenever possible, take on home improvement projects such as painting and wallpapering by yourself. You'll get a workout and save money, says Pierson.

Keep moving. Take 5 minutes here and there throughout the day to play a game with yourself: Do anything except sit or lie down, says Peggy Norwood, former director of the fitness program at Duke University and president of

Playing tennis. Doubles doesn't count unless you play vigorously. Opt for singles matches more often, or at least volunteer to chase a lot of balls.

Cheering your kids' baseball team. Watching a game makes you a loyal fan, not a physically active parent. Walk around the ball field or volunteer to be a referee or a coach to improve your aerobic effort.

Running errands. Your errands probably mean walking from your house to your car. When you can, leave your car in one centralized spot and walk to, from, and between as many places as you can.

Watching the kids. Too many adults sit on a park bench or sofa while their kids run free. Join in the fun.

Housekeeping. Although maintaining a house takes a lot of time, most chores don't make you fit. Put more oomph into it and mop, scrub, vacuum, and sweep with vigor.

Avalon Fitness, both in Durham, North Carolina. Walk out to your garden and check the tomatoes, for example, or carry some clutter up to the attic. Empty the dishwasher. Pace the floor while you talk on the phone.

Hide the remote control. Without a remote control, you have to get up and walk to the television to change the channel. You also may watch less television, says Norwood.

Pull up short. When you are taking a cab, allow some extra time and have the driver drop you off a few blocks away from your destination. If you're taking a bus, get off a stop or two before you need to, then walk.

Run with the dogs. If you're the proud owner of a sprightly canine, you know your pup is happy to go out anytime. Give in to the eager pleading in those friendly eyes. The more you walk your pet, the more excess fat you lose.

Lunch away. Walk somewhere at least 5 minutes from your work area to eat your lunch. After eating, return by a roundabout route so you enjoy a 10-minute walk.

Take exercise breaks. During breaks at work, walk the stairs or walk around the building instead of reading the paper or visiting the watercooler, says Pierson.

Hike to the rest room. Start using a bathroom on a different floor than the one on which you work, or at least use one that is farther away from your office, says Mangan.

Get That Extra Burn

When it comes to burning calories, every little bit counts. Here are 50 ways to burn an extra 150.

1. Iron clothes for 68 minutes.
2. Shoot pool for 58 minutes.
3. Canoe leisurely for 50 minutes.
4. Cook for 48 minutes.
5. Wash and wax a car for 45 to 60 minutes.
6. Wash windows or floors for 45 to 60 minutes.
7. Paper a wall for 45 minutes.
8. Play volleyball for 45 minutes.
9. Ballroom dance for 43 minutes.
10. Stock shelves for 40 minutes.
11. Play croquet for 38 minutes.
12. Reel in a large, feisty fish for 36 minutes.
13. Mop floors for 36 minutes.
14. Grocery shop for 36 minutes.
15. Walk moderately for 1¾ miles in 35 minutes.
16. Dust for 34 minutes.
17. Vacuum for 34 minutes.

18. Play horseshoes for 33 minutes.
19. Play table tennis for 33 minutes.
20. Garden for 30 to 45 minutes.
21. Wheel yourself in a wheelchair for 30 to 45 minutes.
22. Do a country line dance for 30 minutes.
23. Shoot baskets for 30 minutes.
24. Bicycle leisurely for 5 miles in 30 minutes.
25. Dance fast for 30 minutes.
26. Push a stroller for 1½ miles in 30 minutes.
27. Rake leaves for 30 minutes.
28. Walk briskly for 2 miles in 30 minutes.
29. Mow the lawn with a power push mower for 29 minutes.
30. Snowmobile for 29 minutes.
31. Golf without a cart for 26 minutes.
32. Inline skate leisurely for 26 minutes.
33. Stack firewood for 25 minutes.
34. Snorkel for 24 minutes.
35. Bowl for 23 minutes.
36. Play badminton for 22 minutes.
37. Play Frisbee for 22 minutes.
38. Scrub floors for 20 minutes.
39. Saw wood by hand for 18 minutes.
40. Skip rope for 18 minutes.
41. Groom a horse for 17 minutes.
42. Backpack with an 11-pound load for 17 minutes.
43. Ride a motorcycle for 16 minutes.
44. Fork hay for 16 minutes.
45. Twirl a baton for 16 minutes.
46. Bicycle fast for 4 miles in 15 minutes.
47. Shovel snow for 15 minutes.
48. Climb stairs for 15 minutes.
49. Do the twist for 13 minutes.
50. Snowshoe in soft snow for 13 minutes.

Put It All Together

Whatever approach you select or whatever combination you choose, keep these guidelines in mind.

Start slowly. Precede each session with at least 5 minutes of gentle warmup that mimics your upcoming aerobic activity or sport, moving at an easy pace. If you stretch, do it gently, without bouncing movements, after your muscles are warmed up. Otherwise you may cause injury to your joints.

Wind down. At the end of each aerobic session, keep moving until your heart rate gradually returns to normal. This cooldown period, however brief, is critical from a health and safety standpoint, Dr. Fiatarone Singh says, because it allows your body to return gradually to its pre-exercise state. Never stop exercising suddenly. After some heat-generating exercise, you may be tempted to come to a standstill, sit down, or start talking to a friend. But don't let anything distract you from a sensible cooldown period of up to 5 minutes.

Use major muscles. To burn more calories, try to do an exercise such as walking, jogging, stairclimbing (without holding on to the rails), using a ski machine, and rowing, which use large muscle groups in both your upper and lower body, says Dr. Fiatarone Singh.

Write it down. We usually overestimate by 50 percent the amount of time we spend exercising, says Susan J. Bartlett, Ph.D., associate director of clinical psychology at the Johns Hopkins Weight Management Center in Baltimore. Tracking the amount of time you spend exercising can help ensure that you are getting in enough activity as well as help you stay motivated.

Crank It Up

Once you make aerobic exercise a habit, you can look for opportunities to burn a few extra calories. Here are some suggestions.

Go longer, faster. When you begin to exercise, starting off slow and easy is prudent. Then, when you're ready for more action and you feel you can keep it up for the rest of your life, go for it. "The more you do, the better off you are," says Adele L. Franks, M.D., scientific editor for the 1996 Surgeon General's report on physical activity and assistant director for science at the National Center for Chronic Disease Prevention and Health Promotion at the CDC. "You can achieve measurable health benefits by exercising moderately for 30 minutes, 5 days a week. But you can get an even greater benefit if you increase the time or the intensity."

Sweat in short bursts. Research shows that high-intensity training, such as sprinting, burns the most calories and also elevates your metabolism for a longer time than lower-intensity activities. If you can increase the intensity a notch or two a few times during your workout, you'll reap increased calorie-burning benefits afterward, says Dr. Fiatarone Singh. So if you're working out on an exercise bike, for instance, cycle as fast as you can for 90 seconds, then slow down, catch your breath, and continue at your normal pace. Then do it again once you feel comfortable.

Stretch your time. "It's known that the only way to maintain weight loss forever is to increase the amount of physical activity you do," says Miriam Nelson, Ph.D., research scientist at the exercise physiology research center at the Jean Mayer USDA Human Nutrition Research Center on Aging at Tufts University. Indeed, a reader survey conducted by *Prevention* magazine found that although people of optimal weight were no more active in their daily lives than overweight respondents, they did participate in more intentional exercise. Most of those in the optimal weight group said their workout sessions lasted between a ½ hour and an hour. Severely overweight respondents most commonly reported the shortest exercise sessions—less than 20 minutes.

Keep the Weight Off

Which is harder, losing 20 pounds in 6 months or keeping it off the following year?

Lots of people would say the first is harder. But the really hard part, experts say, is *staying* slim. Of those millions of overweight Americans who manage to lose weight, 40 to 60 percent regain it within a year. Others are luckier: They may have up to 5 years before all the pounds pile back on.

"Losing fat and keeping it off in the long term is difficult for many people, but it's by far one of the most important things you can do for your health," says Roger G. Sargent, Ph.D., professor of public health and nutrition at the University of South Carolina School of Public Health in Columbia.

Healing Moves

Despite the health benefits of staying trim, most people tend to overlook exercise as their number one weapon in the lifelong fight against fat. You know you should exercise. Often, you even plan to exercise. But in the hectic crush of day-to-day commitments, it's easy to just skip it.

Don't overlook the obvious. While exercise may seem like just another obligation in an already complicated life, it's a critical part of any long-term strategy you take to lose weight, says Art Mollen, D.O., director of the Southwest Health Institute in Phoenix and author of *Run for Your Life* and *The Mollen Method*. "If you want to fight fat long-term, you must exercise long-term," he says. "Do you eat every day? Of course. If you're putting energy into your system, you need to take energy out of it to maintain your weight."

Wayne C. Miller, Ph.D., assistant professor of kinesiology at Indiana University in Bloomington and director of the university's weight-loss clinic, agrees. "Anything can help you lose weight, but research shows that people who want to keep the weight off need to exercise."

Make Health Your Hobby

Don't you wish you could approach exercise and weight loss with the same zeal you bring to your hobbies? Unfortunately, we tend to view exercise as being a dull or unfulfilling part of life. But there are ways to bring to exercise and fitness the same vigor you bring to your play.

Follow your heart. The best exercise for long-term weight control isn't the one that makes you sweat the most. It's the one you'll actually do, be it golf, aerobics, gardening, or swimming.

"You don't get people to change to a healthy lifestyle by boring them. You have to make exercise fun," says Joan Price, a fitness instructor and owner of Unconventional Moves, a fitness consulting service in Sebastopol, California.

Get involved. Serious hobbyists get nearly fanatical when it comes to pursuing the minutiae of their interests, which is why they stick with them year after year. To turn an exercise habit into a hobby, get involved. No matter what you like, somewhere there's a newspaper, magazine, or newsletter that covers it. Check your local newsstand or magazine rack. If you can't find what you're looking for, ask your librarian for help.

Join your peers. Joining a club with like-minded fitness buffs is a great way to keep in long-term shape, says Price. You'll make new friends, have a regular group to hang out with, and get someone who'll push you to work out on days when you'd rather slump.

Diversify. When you make exercise or sports your hobby, it's like being part of a family, says Price. That means sharing similarities and differences. "For example, if you're both cyclists and your new friend likes to play tennis, try it. You might pick up another hobby, and at the very least, you'll be getting more exercise and broadening your horizons."

Creative Tricks for Staying in Shape

It's easy to talk about exercise as a way to stay in shape, but it's a lot harder to actually get around to doing it. Or is it?

Not necessarily. You don't even have to do sports, lift weights, or sweat to music. "You need to work fat off any way you can, so the more creative your solution, the better," says Steven N. Blair, director of epidemiology and clinical applications at the Cooper Institute for Aerobics Research in Dallas. "I suspect the traditional advice, like exercising three times a week for 30 minutes, is good for some people, but I'm not convinced that it's the best approach for everybody."

In one study, researchers divided overweight kids into three groups. Kids in one group did a prescribed amount and type of exercise. Those in the second group were allowed to choose their activity, while kids in the third group did regular calisthenics and stretching. After 8 weeks, children in all groups lost about the same amount of weight. But in a 2-year follow-up, it was the ones who had chosen their activities, like walking to and from school, who managed to keep the weight off.

"The bottom line is, you need to increase your physical activity any way you can; do something rather than nothing," Dr. Blair says.

Here are some creative approaches to staying thin year after year.

Control the remote. If you spend every night clicking away the channels with a remote control, don't be surprised when you start resembling sofa sediment with a paunch. "The technology revolution is such that it's engineered physical activity right out of our lifestyle," Dr. Blair says. "We can do so much nowadays without even moving."

That's the trend, but it's easy to reverse. Just losing the remote control can help. Take those few extra steps across the living room and change the channels yourself. Doing this several times an hour will burn more calories than lying still, and every little bit helps.

Take to the streets. You don't have to be a runner to put your legs in motion. If you live reasonably close to work, for instance, try leaving the car parked and hoof it instead. Walking an hour at a leisurely 3.5 miles an hour will burn about 300 calories.

Too far to walk? Try cycling. An increasing number of people are two-wheeling their way to work every day, burning about 650 calories an hour while cruising along at 13 miles an hour.

Time to Get Personal

When you need an extra boost, consider signing up with a personal trainer. You'll get personalized attention, plus you'll be able to work at your pace. And a trainer's rates aren't necessarily out of reach. Most charge between $30 and $200 for a 50-minute session. The rate may include the use of a local gym or health club, or the trainer may work with you at home. But before making the hire, here's what experts suggest.

Cast a wide network. You can always peruse the yellow pages, but a better idea is to ask your friends and coworkers if they know anyone. Or ask around at the health club.

Look for longevity. Ask prospective trainers how long they've been in business and what their experience is. You're looking for seasoned pros, not beginners trying to break into a new profession.

Ask about credentials. The oldest and most reputable programs that certify trainers are the American College of Sports Medicine, the National Academy of Sports Medicine, and the National Strength and Conditioning Association. Other good programs include the Cooper Institute for Aerobics Research, the American Council on Exercise, and the Aerobics and Fitness Association of America.

Request references. Good trainers have satisfied customers with whom they won't hesitate to put you in touch. Ask to speak to three.

Take a trial run. Before signing up for a long-term program, arrange a 1-month trial period. How well you get along with this person will really determine whether you stick with the program. If it's not a good match, cut your losses and move on.

Make the most of vacations. It's hard to think of anything negative to say about spending a week on a sandy Mexican beach. Suffice it to say that it won't help your waist get any smaller. In fact, after a few days of margaritas and rich food, you can expect it to be *mucho grande* by the time you say adios.

A fun alternative to the usual lounge about is to take an exercise vacation, a few days or weeks in which you put your muscles to work instead of to bed. Rather than tanning on the beach in Cancún, for example, you could be cycling through the countryside in Mexico or here in the United States—take your pick. Even spinning at a moderate pace of 10 miles an hour will burn about 400 calories an hour.

Get Pumping

Anytime the talk turns to losing weight and keeping it off, you're going to hear about the two cornerstones of exercise: aerobic activities and resistance training.

Aerobic exercises are those that make your body demand oxygen and burn calories, like walking, running, rowing, aerobic dancing, or any other moderate-to-vigorous physical activity. Resistance training (weight lifting), on the other hand, is anaerobic exercise, which builds muscle mass through resistance.

Whichever workout you choose, here are a few steps to make it most efficient.

Don't lie to yourself. "Understand that some goals are achievable and others are pipe dreams," Dr. Blair says. "We all come in different shapes and sizes. I've come to grips with the fact that I'll never look like a movie star, no matter how much I run."

Lift for life. You probably haven't seen many 70-year-olds pumping iron at the local gym, but you might in the future. That's because experts are now realizing that weight lifting is the unsung hero of fat-fighting exercises, says Dr. Sargent.

"I feel that the only reason resistance training hasn't had the same glory attached to it as aerobics is that it hasn't had as much study," Dr. Sargent says. "You'll find, in the past 5 to 6 years, that the results of weight-loss studies on resistance training and aerobics have been fairly equivalent." While advanced lifters can spend hours pumping iron, 20 to 30 minutes is enough for most people.

As you get stronger and more experienced, you may want to start experimenting with different lifting styles: lifting light weights with higher repetitions, or going for more weight with fewer reps. According to Dr. Sargent, evidence suggests lifting light weights, more often, yields greater muscle strength than using heavier weights. Regardless of the strategy you choose, lifting weights increases muscle mass, which ups your metabolism and helps you burn fat more efficiently.

Go aerobic. If experts could choose just one type of exercise to rout that Rubenesque look, they'd choose aerobic exercise, roughly defined as any exercise that increases your consumption of oxygen, causing your heart rate to increase.

These days there are more aerobic options than New York City has pizza joints: running, cycling, rowing, skiing, boxing, wrestling, basketball, walking—all of which can provide a fantastic aerobic workout.

The American College of Sports Medicine and the federal Centers for Disease Control and Prevention recommend doing 30 minutes of moderate-intensity activity, such as walking or running, every day. It doesn't have to be done all at once, however. Rather, it can be accumulated with small amounts of activity scattered throughout the day.

"For real results, you're going to have to work at it," notes Dr. Mollen. While you may choose to start out doing 30 minutes of exercise seven times a week, eventually you'll want to bump your times to 45 to 60 minutes daily, he says.

Team up with team sports. Not everyone wants to be a lonely marathoner treading for hours in self-imposed solitude. Some of us want to shoot the breeze while we're sweating away the pounds. For both the workout and the social fun, team sports are ideal.

If you don't already have a network of friends active on a variety of playing fields, check the newspaper for sports leagues near you. A spot on the community softball team or bowling league might be all you need to stick to a life-long exercise regimen.

If you strike out at finding an established community league, start a game yourself by recruiting in the office. Your coworkers might jump at the chance for some high-noon athletic antics.

PART FOUR

Think Yourself Thin

Stop Eating
for the Wrong Reasons

Name a feeling, and most of us can name the food that goes with it. Angry? Maybe you turn to potato chips. Sad? Ice cream is the perfect antidote. Joyful? Nothing satisfies like pizza.

Why do you turn to food when moodiness strikes? Most likely, you can blame it on your parents and your pediatrician. When you were an infant, your parents fed you whenever you cried. As a young tyke, you might have been offered a chocolate bar after you skinned your knee. Or perhaps you always got a lollipop after braving a booster shot. And you got to celebrate good report cards and sporting triumphs with trips to the local pizza joint.

Even if you were never rewarded with food, though, you probably figured out its healing emotional nature on your own. Fat- and sugar-laden treats taste good and feel good in our mouths, providing instant pleasure that elevates a bad mood, if only for a few fleeting moments, says Dianne Lindewall, Ph.D., supervising behavioral psychologist with the George Washington University Obesity

Management Program in Washington, D.C. "On that level, it's hard for a carrot to compete with a bowl of ice cream," she says.

Also, foods like ice cream, cakes, and candy are rich in carbohydrates and so may elevate levels of a feel-good brain chemical called serotonin, temporarily boosting your sense of well-being, says Dr. Lindewall.

For women, this carbohydrate connection may be especially strong during the second half of the menstrual cycle, after ovulation. At that time, progesterone levels rise, causing a drop in blood sugar and increased food cravings, says Elizabeth Lee Vliet, M.D., founder and medical director of HER Place: Health Enhancement and Renewal for Women, a women's center in Tucson; and author of *Screaming to Be Heard: Hormonal Connections Women Suspect . . . and Doctors Ignore.*

Snipping the Food/Mood Link

It's okay to turn to chocolate chip cookies occasionally. But if we turn to pistachio fudge and marble pound cake to soothe our everyday disappointments, we're headed for trouble, says Linda Smolak, Ph.D., professor of psychology at Kenyon College in Gambier, Ohio. Habitually seeking solace with rich comfort foods can lead to overweight. Here's how to hold off the pounds no matter how bad the emotional crisis.

Don't deny yourself completely. You're more likely to turn to food for comfort if your diet leaves you feeling deprived, says Dr. Smolak. Studies show that restrained eaters, those who diet or strictly control food intake to maintain a low weight, seem especially susceptible to responding to strong feelings by reaching for something to eat. If you want to slim down, don't crash diet.

Keep a food/mood journal. Jot your thoughts in a pocket-size notebook, in your day planner, or on a 3-by-5 card. Answer the following questions.

- Am I physically hungry?
- What do I want to eat?
- What am I feeling?
- What am I saying to myself?
- Who is with me?
- What has been going on in the past hours or the past day?

Pause before you eat, and identify your true needs—emotional or physical hunger, says Donna Ciliska, R.N., Ph.D., associate professor of health sciences at McMaster University in Hamilton, Ontario, and author of *Beyond Dieting*. "Once you identify your emotions, the long-term goal is finding new ways to cope." Keep the journal for a week, review your notes, and search for your emotional-eating triggers.

Find solutions that don't involve food. Once you've identified a situation that makes you turn to food for comfort, you need to come up with a different response. If your boss makes you feel unappreciated, think about strategies to deal with it that don't involve eating.

Share your feelings. Tell your children, your partner, and your close friends about the positive feelings you have for them, says Gail Post, Ph.D., a clinical psychologist in Jenkintown, Pennsylvania. Don't rely on making them a batch of cookies or taking them out for pizza to express how you feel.

Seek out support. Sometimes, the problem is that there's no one you can talk to. If loneliness drives you to eat, a support group like Overeaters Anonymous can be helpful. Even if there is someone to talk to at home, it's

The Best (and Worst) Mood Foods

Regardless of whether we're celebrating a job promotion, lamenting a romance on the rocks, or fervently plotting the downfall of a rival, we usually reach for something that's loaded with fat and calories. Yet we could easily satisfy our moody yearnings with healthier alternatives, says Susan Olson, Ph.D., a clinical psychologist and weight-management consultant in Seattle and author of *Keeping It Off: Winning at Weight Loss*. When various moods strike, here's what we eat and why—and what to grab instead.

Anger and Stress

What we usually eat: Potato chips, corn chips, or nuts

Why: Crunching hard foods releases aggression and tension in the jaw

Better alternatives: Sugarless gum, pretzels, carrots, or low-fat crackers

Sadness, a Broken Heart, or Depression

What we usually eat: Chocolate, ice cream, or cheese

Why: The smooth consistency soothes us. Chemically, chocolate contains a mood-elevating substance that acts like an antidepressant

Better alternatives: Nonfat chocolate frozen yogurt, hot chocolate, or vegetable soup

Happiness

What we usually eat: Pizza, chips with dip, or cake

Why: Traditionally, we associate such foods with celebrations

Better alternatives: Vegetarian pizza without cheese, shrimp cocktail, or watermelon

often easier to discuss difficult circumstances with people who share them, says Dr. Smolak.

Treat yourself well. Instead of reaching for food, take a walk, soak in a warm tub, play your favorite CD, call a friend, work on your hobby, or relax with a new book.

Use self-talk. Words are powerful. By repeating an affirmation that focuses on the solutions you can use instead of overeating when you feel unloved, you actually make it less likely that you'll turn to the pantry for nurturing, says Nan Kathryn Fuchs, Ph.D., a nutritionist in Sebastopol, California, and author of *Overcoming the Legacy of Overeating*. Try repeating the following statements for 5 to 10 minutes every day: "I handle my problems well. I eat food to nourish myself." Or come up with your own affirmation. Put it in the present tense, even if it is not what you are now doing. In time, you will do it.

Encourage yourself. Throughout the day, listen to how your self-talk is going, suggests Barbara Dickinson, R.D., director of nutrition at the weight-management center at Loma Linda University in California. Is your inner voice critical, self-defeating, or full of commands? Counter negative messages with truthful, positive responses. Turn a comment like "I can't talk with my new coworkers; they won't like me," for example, into "I'd like to get to know them better; I'll begin with some questions about our office during coffee break."

Put moods in perspective. "Tell yourself, 'This feeling will pass whether I eat or not,'" says psychotherapist Mary Anne Cohen, director of the New York Center for Eating Disorders in New York City. Sometimes, people cannot tolerate discomfort because they think it will last forever. You need to realize that feelings have a beginning, a middle, and an end.

Solve the problem. What's prompting you to reach for food at the moment? A work deadline? A conflict with your spouse? Try to focus on solving the problem, rather than distract yourself with food. If the issue cannot be resolved immediately, write the solution down and get on with your day.

Take a time-out. For 10 minutes, resist the urge to nosh and ask yourself what's going on. Figure out what's behind that craving, says Sandra Campbell, Psy.D., clinical director of the eating disorders program at the Brattleboro Retreat in Vermont. And make it a habit to tune in to your inner feelings at these times.

"Sometimes, you just need a few minutes to pull yourself together," says Susan Moore, R.D., program manager and senior nutritionist with the George Washington University Obesity Management Program.

Reach out and call someone. A brief phone call to a friend or relative may distract you and provide the emotional connection you really crave, says Connie Roberts, R.D., manager of nutrition consultation services and wellness programs at Brigham and Women's Hospital in Boston. "You don't have to tell them you were about to eat four chocolate cupcakes," she says. "Just chat. It helps."

Delay. Come up in advance with a list of alternative activities to do when the eating mood strikes. At work, tack the list to your calendar. It could include reading your mail or the newspaper. At home, sew a button on that shirt that's been out of commission for months. Polish the car or your shoes. Repot your favorite fern.

Practice safe snacking. We all need an emotional pick-me-up once in a while. Try satisfying your need with tasty foods in small portions. This approach also keeps you from fearing the foods you desire. "I have patients practice buying one chocolate truffle and enjoying it to the utmost," says Roberts. "Sometimes, denying yourself the one thing you want can lead to eating more calories somewhere else."

Plan. If you must eat, tell yourself in advance what snacks you'll turn to when emotion-driven episodes occur, says Roberts. Possible examples include air-popped popcorn or a muffin.

Nurture yourself. Take care of yourself, suggests Dr. Ciliska. You may need more rest, more creative and intellectual stimulation, or the opportunity to express your feelings and be heard. You may need new sources of comfort, nurturing, and love, which could range from setting aside time for a relaxing bath or listening to your favorite music to developing new friendships.

Speak your mind. If you stuff down anger, learning to ask assertively for what you need can help, Dr. Ciliska says. This may require taking an assertiveness training class, she says.

"I don't know any people, myself included, who haven't benefited from some assertiveness training," notes Dr. Lindewall. "Learning to speak up for yourself without being timid or intimidating is a very important skill."

Make time for simply doing nothing. Are you stressed? Are mealtimes and snack times the only times you allow yourself to relax? If so, you may be eating just to get a breather from a nonstop routine, notes Susan Irish-Zelener, Psy.D., a clinical psychologist at the Center for Health Promotion at Loma Linda University. "A lot of people feel tremendous guilt if they stop working for even a minute," she says. "You work hard all day, eat lunch at your desk, and then spend the evening doing chores. You may have a snack or spend a long time over dinner because, for most of us, it's the only time that we give ourselves permission to stop working." Instead, take the time to listen to music, read, watch a movie, or simply not do anything at all, she says.

Put some excitement in your life. Are you bored? Thinking of perking up a dull day with chocolate-covered cherries? Don't. Instead, seek new job challenges, revive a long-lost hobby, or find a new one, suggests Dr. Ciliska. "I've known people to ask their supervisors for more di-

Do Your Emotions Drive Your Eating Habits?

Getting a handle on emotional eating is the very first step toward successful weight control, says Ronette Kolotkin, Ph.D., director of the behavioral program at the Duke University Diet and Fitness Center in Durham, North Carolina, and coauthor of *The Duke University Medical Center Book of Diet and Fitness*. How can you tell if you are an emotional eater? Answer yes or no to the following statements, then check your score below.

1. I often eat for reasons other than hunger.
2. When I am overwhelmed, I often eat to find relief.
3. I usually eat to calm myself down.
4. When I am angry, I turn to food.
5. Whenever things feel out of control, I eat more.
6. If someone dislikes me or puts me down, I often turn to food to feel better.
7. When I'm happy, eating makes me feel happier.
8. When I want to reward myself, I eat.
9. Food is more than nutritional fuel. It's my best friend, my comforter, my escape, a source of unconditional love.
10. If I'm lonely or bored, I overeat and feel better.

If you answered yes to five or six of the statements, food is moderately important in your emotional life, says Dr. Kolotkin. If you have seven or more yes answers, food has a central role in your emotional life. You may eat to avoid unpleasant feelings or as a substitute for love, intimacy, achievement, or even fun. Keeping a food/mood diary and using other tactics to prevent emotional-eating episodes may help you meet those needs.

verse job responsibilities," she says. "If you feel bored at home, think about past activities you've enjoyed, such as a sport or a handicraft." Or peruse the community calendar of your local newspaper for new activities, from volunteer opportunities and quilting circles to tennis classes and wildflower-identification walks.

Eat every 4 hours. Skimping on breakfast and lunch can leave you hungry, irritable, and vulnerable to emotional eating, says Dickinson. The antidote is to eat the right foods, at the right times. Most people find that a substantial breakfast that totals about 400 calories is helpful. Include a protein food (such as 2%, 1%, or fat-free milk or low-fat or nonfat yogurt or cottage cheese), grains (like whole wheat toast, oatmeal, or a high-fiber cereal), and fruit, says Dickinson. "Plan on eating lunch 4 hours later and dinner 4 hours after that," she says. It's also good to include a small amount of a healthy fat in your meals, from avocado, peanut butter, nuts, canola oil, or olive oil. These fats, comprised largely of monounsaturated and polyunsaturated fats, help you feel satisfied.

Do something with your hands. For some people, unwinding with food can easily be replaced by gardening, a craft, or even computer games—anything that involves fine-motor movement of the fingers and hands," says Irish. Somehow, small, repeated movements help us chill out after a long day.

Figure out what you want. If you've paused and still want to nosh, think of ways to minimize the binge. Before you grab a candy bar or a big slice of cake, be clear about the food experience you're seeking, says Moore. "Find out what you really want," she says. "Will a cup of coffee do, or do you really need a candy bar? Are you looking for a specific taste, or do you want to fill yourself up? If it's a special taste, then maybe a small candy bar is all you need. If it's volume you're after, maybe fruit or popcorn is a smart choice."

Bargain down the size. Once you've decided what you want, ask yourself how much you really need, says Moore. Half a candy bar or a whole one? Will half a piece of cake satisfy you? "By keeping the size down, maybe to just a taste, you control overeating," she says.

Interrupt yourself before the next bite. If you find yourself on automatic pilot, mindlessly reaching into the cookie bag, stop for a moment. "Ask yourself if this is really what you want to be doing and if there is anything else you'd rather be doing instead," suggests Dickinson. "Often, emotional eating is done quickly. You don't realize what's going on until the food is all gone. Pause and be aware."

Balance the calories. Think about how much your indulgence will cost in terms of calories, then plan accordingly. You can compensate for the extra calories that come with an episode of emotional eating by eating less at another meal or two or by getting more physical activity, says Moore. Compensating for a 250-calorie chocolate bar, for example, would mean skipping bread and butter at dinner and walking an extra mile. "If you think about balancing the calories ahead of time, you might decide that the candy bar just isn't worth it," Moore says.

Defuse high-risk times. Your mother is coming for a visit? Almost time for the annual family holiday gathering and all the tense moments that come with it? "If you can predict high-risk situations and get ready for them, you can balance out the added calories in some way," Dr. Lindewall says. "You can always eat a little less before and afterward."

Challenge all-or-nothing thinking. If you do find yourself crunching instead of coping, don't despair. "That doesn't make you a bad person or mean that you've ruined everything," says Dickinson. "Even if you still experience some overeating, remember that you're making a change. It takes time. Don't lose sight of that."

The Real Reason
That Diets Fail

Stress—it's so familiar, you can taste it. Inside your body, your adrenal glands start pumping out the hormones epinephrine and norepinephrine, which tense up your muscles and speed up your heart rate and breathing and raise your blood pressure. And you're as jumpy as a cat in a car wash.

A few thousand years ago, such tensed muscles and a palpitating heart would have helped you run a few hundred yards in record time, hopefully fast enough to escape being gored to death by some really big, hairy animal with sharp fangs.

Today, such a sensation makes you reach for a dozen or so chocolate chunk cookies or some other majorly fattening comfort food. In today's world, stress and weight gain go hand in hand.

Soothing Solutions

Here's how to get that fattening stress monkey off your back.

Take a moment to relax. Stress is most damaging if it's unrelenting. Just a few moments of relaxation can help considerably, says Susan Heitler, Ph.D., a clinical psychologist in Denver and author of the audiotape *Anxiety: Friend or Foe?* "Take mini-breaks," she says. "If you're at work and you start feeling stressed, get up and stretch or talk to a coworker for a couple of minutes." If you're home, take a break in a quiet room.

Give yourself a longer break at least once every day, says Sharon Greenburg, Ph.D., a clinical psychologist in private practice in Chicago.

Talk it out. If you have more to do than you can realistically handle or too little control over your schedule to get things done, speak up, says Deborah Belle, Ed.D., associate professor of psychology at Boston University. At work, talk to your boss. She may have no idea that you are overloaded or that your assignments are so ambiguous that you spend an extra hour each day trying to figure out what's expected, she says. Or consult coworkers to find out if and how they've handled similar situations.

"If nothing else, you'll feel less powerless because you've spoken up, and that sense of control can significantly reduce the negative impact of stress," says Dr. Heitler.

At home, talk to your spouse. "In relationships, poor communication is often the source of stress," says Rosalind Barnett, Ph.D., senior scientist in the women's studies program at Brandeis University in Waltham, Massachusetts, and coauthor of *She Works, He Works*.

Go easy on yourself. "If you're in a job where expectations are unrealistic, you'll only feel more stressed if you tell yourself, 'I'm really incompetent,'" says Dr. Greenburg. "Instead, be objective. Tell yourself, 'I'm doing as much as anyone could, and more.'"

At home, accept the fact that you can't give the people you love everything, says Dr. Barnett. "So do the best job you can and be okay with that."

Off-load some chores. Women who work full-time outside the home still do more than half of the housework, especially tasks such as grocery shopping, meal preparation and cleanup, and child-oriented duties such as bathing and helping with homework, studies show. Strive for a more even split. Your husband actually may enjoy some of his new responsibilities. "Our research finds that, for many husbands, being with the kids actually feels like a reward after a hard day at the office," says Dr. Barnett. "When husbands and wives share more equally, everyone feels less stress."

Think before you cut. Many people assume that all of their obligations add more stress, says Dr. Belle. "But research actually suggests that people with many roles—worker, parent, spouse, community volunteer—fare better," she says. Evidently, the satisfaction you get from one role can buffer the stress that you feel in another. So before you give up your post as a Scout leader, ask yourself what you're getting out of it, says Dr. Belle. It may be providing leadership opportunities that are lacking at work, for example. By the same token, the sense of satisfaction and mastery that you get at work could be the ideal antidote to the stress you feel while raising a teenager. More roles may also mean a wider stress-relieving social support network.

Exercise. The feeling of well-being that you get from physical activity can counter pressure both at home and at the office, says Camille Lloyd, Ph.D., professor in the department of psychiatry and behavioral sciences at the University of Texas–Houston Medical School. Activities that get you moving, such as tennis, volleyball, running, swimming, or walking, are ideal because they burn off stress-related chemicals. They also strengthen your heart so that it can withstand the future ravages of stress.

Pop bubbles. One study found that students were able to reduce their feelings of tension by popping two sheets of those plastic air capsules used in packaging. "Now we know why people hoard those things," says Kathy M. Dillon, Ph.D., professor of psychology at Western New England College in Springfield, Massachusetts, and author of the study.

Carry a humor first-aid kit. Laughter can change your mood and take you out of an eating frame of mind, says Linda Welsh, Ed.D., director of the Agoraphobia and Anxiety Treatment Center in Bala Cynwyd, Pennsylvania. "You're changing your brain chemistry and putting yourself in an altered state," she says. "It works physically as well as emotionally in that it lets go of the tension and improves your outlook." Watch a funny movie or read a humorous book, she suggests.

Stop and smell the apples. Keeping a green apple on your desk may calm your nerves. Research shows that the scent of the apple can significantly reduce stress and anxiety levels.

Think twice about caffeine. Some studies show that a little caffeine can increase alertness. But drinking coffee, tea, or other caffeinated beverages is apt to leave you feeling jittery and irritable in the long run, says Georgia Hodgkin, R.D., Ed.D., associate professor in the department of nutrition and dietetics at Loma Linda University in California.

In fact, researchers at Duke University in Durham, North Carolina, have found that caffeine can actually stimulate the body's fight-or-flight response to stress.

Keep your hands out of the sugar bowl. Too much sugar robs your body of vital nutrients, causing nervous tension and anxiety. It also fuels the fight-or-flight response, which overworks your adrenal glands and triggers vasoconstriction, or narrowing of the blood vessels, further contributing to stress. High-sugar foods also make blood sugar levels rise, promoting an infusion of insulin, which ushers the sugar into your cells, which in turn drops blood sugar levels, says Dr. Hodgkin. "When blood sugar levels

One More Reason to De-Stress

Even if you manage to avoid fatty, sugary foods when stress knocks on your door, you could still gain weight. Stress seems to encourage your body to store fat, regardless of your eating and exercise habits. It triggers a starvation response, an unconscious tendency to conserve energy from food as if your body were preparing for famine. So when stress hormones begin coursing through your body, you start storing calories as fat. Also, during stress, blood sugar is shunted away from the chemical pathways that would burn it, so instead of being burned for fuel, it is stored as fat.

To avoid the fat–stress connection, you need to do more than practice good eating and exercise habits: You need to learn to cope with stress. That's why breathing techniques and other relaxation exercises are so important.

drop, you can feel irritable, tired, and unhappy, which is the last thing you need under stress," she says.

Plan for snack attacks. If you snack, avoid high-fat, high-calorie snack-machine fare by eating your own treats, says Dr. Hodgkin. Stock a desk drawer with apples and oranges, low-fat microwave popcorn, or single-serving boxes of crunchy, low-sugar cereal.

Delay. Do you crave a packet of chocolate-covered raisins when a deadline looms? Wait 10 minutes, and the urge may pass, says Carla Wolper, R.D., nutritionist and clinical coordinator at the obesity research center at St. Luke's–Roosevelt Hospital Center in New York City. "Or have a nice cup of caffeine-free tea. Or take a short break. Distracting yourself for 10 minutes could be all you need," she says.

Decide what you can deal with and forget the rest. List the most stressful situations in your life. Then list the ones you can change (like leaving late for work in the morning) and the ones you can't (like getting caught in the daily traffic jam at the toll booth). Prioritize the ones you can control, then outline a de-stressing action plan.

Defuse. Even when you're pressed for time, you can take 3 minutes to defuse a stressful situation and derail the need to eat, says Ronette Kolotkin, Ph.D., director of the

Take a Deep Breath

Proper breathing is one of the most effective ways to lower stress levels and head off stress-induced feeding frenzies.

"People who are stressed don't breathe properly," says Martha Davis, Ph.D., who teaches relaxation training at Kaiser Permanente Medical Center in Santa Clara, California. "To demonstrate this, I'll often ask my students to follow my finger as I wave it back and forth in front of their eyes. Then I'll ask how many of them stopped breathing. If they're honest and paying attention, most will realize that they stopped breathing for a few seconds. If they stopped breathing with something as mundane as my waving my finger, how often do all of us stop breathing during the more stressful moments in our lives?"

That's where breathing exercises come in. If you practice breathing on a regular basis, you'll train yourself to breathe deeply and calmly when you encounter any stressful situation. Here are a few exercises to try.

- Lie on your back on the floor. Place your left hand over your chest and your right hand over your belly button. Without consciously altering your breathing,

behavioral program at the Duke University Diet and Fitness Center and coauthor of *The Duke University Medical Center Book of Diet and Fitness*. Step outside for some fresh air. Close your office door and stamp your feet, punch a pillow, or turn on a relaxation tape for a few minutes.

Balance thinking and feeling. Under stress, our conscious selves may recognize that we're not at fault or not in trouble, but our emotional selves may not, says Sylvia Gearing, Ph.D., a clinical psychologist in Dallas and coau-

notice which hand moves. If your right hand rises first and falls last with each breath, that's great. You're breathing with your diaphragm, which is how it should be. An ideal breath should fill the bottom third of your lungs first, then the middle third, and finally the top third, in one smooth motion. If when you do the exercise, your left hand rises first or more than your right hand, you're a shallow chest breather.

• Lie on the floor with a book on your stomach. Concentrate on making the book rise and fall with each breath. Alternately, lie on your stomach and concentrate on pushing your belly against the floor with each inhalation. This exercise will train you to belly breathe.

• Breathe in deeply for a count of four, pause, then breathe out for a count of five. Do this for 3 to 5 minutes; it will have a tranquilizing effect on your body and mind. Counting keeps your breath regulated and gives your mind something to concentrate on.

thor of *Female Executive Stress Syndrome*. "There may be some feelings stirring around in there that you can't calm," she says. "Remind yourself that this will pass, that it will be over soon. Continuing to obsess will not help; it only takes energy away from doing what you have to do."

Get your daily requirement of play. Unwind, suggests Connie Roberts, R.D., manager of nutrition consultation services and wellness programs at Brigham and Women's Hospital in Boston. Set aside playtime. "Go to an art museum, see a movie, or take a walk with a friend," she says.

Know your trigger points. The ultimate stress-control strategy is to know yourself, says Dr. Kolotkin. "Look for patterns," she says. "If you start crying every Sunday night and find you're eating all night long, it could very well be that you're having some feelings about your job and things aren't right. Sometimes, you have to either accept that this is a stressful job and find less stressful work, or take steps to make the job more tolerable. The same is true of relationships. Ultimately, you have two choices: change the situation or accept it."

Take a hike. Regular walking is one way to attack all of your symptoms at once: It can help you lose weight, give you the perfect opportunity to sort out goals and priorities, and reduce stress in a big way.

Put time on your side. Stressed-out people often seem overwhelmed because they're disorganized. They're the ones who don't start making the kids' Halloween costumes until the night before. They also tend to apply equal vigor to every task, even though some tasks are more important than others, and so they feel out of control—a leading cause of workplace anxiety.

If you recognize the symptoms of disorganization in your habits at home and on the job, come up with a system to keep track of your tasks. You might use a notebook, for example. Make a list of everything you need to do and check off each item as you go along. The most pressing tasks go at the top and the least time sensitive go toward the bottom.

List your de-stressors. Plan your bad-mood strategy by making a mental or written list of pleasurable activities. The next time you feel stressed out, for instance, try calling a friend, reading a book, taking a bath, going to the gym, writing your feelings in a journal, playing with your kids or your dog, getting a massage, going to a movie, taking a walk, buying flowers, listening to music, taking a nap, doing volunteer work, visiting a neighbor, taking a yoga class, meditating, or praying.

Listen to music. Music can produce the most profound states of mental and physical relaxation. "In fact, the right music in the hands of a trained music therapist can yield reductions in blood pressure, heart rate, and even the levels of stress hormones, such as cortisol, that the body produces," says Cheryl Dileo, Ph.D., past president of the World Federation of Music Therapy and professor of music therapy at Temple University in Philadelphia.

Listen to your heart. In a study at Tufts University in Boston, 22 middle-aged women who were highly anxious spent 10 minutes a day simply paying attention to their heart rates, using wireless monitors. At the end of 12 weeks, their anxiety levels had dropped to normal. You don't need a monitor to get the same effect. You can listen to your breathing instead. Sit in a quite place and close your eyes. Observe yourself inhaling and exhaling. Don't try to slow your breath or make it deeper; just let it be natural. Focus on the sensation of breath as it passes through your nostrils or the back of your throat. Practice anywhere from 2 to 20 minutes a day.

Eat in the morning. Stress levels rise when your body is low on fuel, says Susan Moore, R.D., program manager and senior nutritionist with the George Washington University Obesity Management Program in Washington,

D.C. "Experiment with a combination of foods until you find out what gives you long-lasting energy," she says. "Some people need more than a bagel and juice; a little protein and fat, like a dab of peanut butter, gives them staying power."

Add a snack. Small pick-me-ups at mid-morning and mid-afternoon can prevent the low energy that leads to anxiety and stress, says Barbara Dickinson, R.D., director of nutrition at the weight-management center at Loma Linda University.

Drink lots of water. Fit in eight glasses (8 ounces each) of water a day, and drink before you get thirsty, Dickinson suggests. Dehydration can cause headaches and fatigue, so you may think you need a snack when all you really need is cool, clear water, she says.

The Most Common Weight-Loss Pitfalls

Do you ever swear off chocolate only to eventually find yourself eating a jumbo bag of M&M's?

Does your mouth say yes while your brain says no every time a coworker brings baked goods to the office?

Do you avoid eating "forbidden foods" in public but then binge on those same foods in private?

Have you quit your weight-loss program because your goal seemed too far away, too hard, even impossible?

If you answered yes to any of these questions, you fall into one or several of the most common weight-loss traps, according to Joyce D. Nash, Ph.D., a clinical psychologist in San Francisco and Palo Alto, California, and author of *The New Maximize Your Body Potential*.

Many times, say psychologists, weight loss fails not only because we are eating too much food or exercising too little but also because we are mentally sabotaging ourselves. The good news is that you can sidestep the sabotage. All you need to do is arm your brain for psychological warfare.

Diversify Your Thinking

Too often, we think in terms of all or nothing. The thought process goes something like this: You tell yourself that you are not allowed to eat chocolate chip cookies. You swear off them. You get through a week, maybe even two, before you see a dozen chocolate chip cookies sitting in the company break room with a large "Free for the taking" sign taped to the box. You take one, then two. Then you tell yourself, "I already messed up. I may as well eat all of them." Then you feel horrible, guilty. And you pledge to never do it again. A week later, you find yourself in the same situation.

Why did you end up eating not one but a dozen cookies? Because your weight-loss plan didn't give you any latitude. Rather than make space for one, two, or even three cookies, you allow yourself none. And when you slip up and have one, you quickly eat all of them while you still can. Such thinking is probably the number-one psychological pitfall of any fat-fighting plan, says Carolyn Costin, director of the Eating Disorders Center of California and the Monte Nido Residential Treatment Center in Malibu and author of *The Eating Disorder Sourcebook* and *Your Dieting Daughter*.

In reality, sometimes you'll stick to your plan, but sometimes you'll overeat. Likewise, sometimes you'll exercise regularly and sometimes you won't. Here are some strategies to pick yourself up, forgive yourself, and keep going.

Avoid making rules. Do any of the following phrases sound familiar?

- "I have to lose 15 pounds before the class reunion."
- "I can't ever snack."
- "I'm giving up chocolate."

If you've made similar resolutions, you're not alone. The trouble is, rigid rules create sabotage traps, says Costin. "The more you deprive yourself of a food, the more you want it," she explains. That's why dieting often fails.

"There's such a big emphasis on resisting food," says Susan Olson, Ph.D., a clinical psychologist and weight-management consultant in Seattle and author of *Keeping It Off: Winning at Weight Loss*. Once you stop following such rules, however, you easily lose weight, she says.

So if you have trouble quitting cold turkey, make sure you have a backup plan. "If you have to set up a rule for yourself, know that you need to be flexible," says Costin. Ask yourself, "If I break this rule, what do I do?" The answer should be "I get back on track."

Imagine a teeter-totter. When you find that you're tottering—maybe you had a lot of fatty foods at dinner—don't make up for it by teetering to the other extreme. Hold your teeter-totter steady; that is, head for balance, says Costin. If you eat a few cookies, for instance, don't resort to eating the whole bag. Also, don't try to make up for it the next day by skipping breakfast. Just start the next day with a clean slate, with your teeter-totter in the center, balanced position, says Costin.

Set realistic expectations. Instead of trying to eat perfectly 100 percent of the time, try to make healthy food choices 80 percent of the time. Then chalk the rest up to human nature, says Dr. Nash.

Give yourself credit. Instead of obsessing about the 1 day out of an entire week that you overate, focus on the 6 that went just fine.

Say No to the Food Pushers

She makes brownies just for you. She stands in your office doorway. You can tell that she won't leave until you try one. So when you eat the brownies, you mentally blame it on her. After all, she talked you into it.

But shifting responsibility to others is flawed thinking.

The food pusher isn't the one who's trying to lose weight or the one who's eating the extra calories. You are.

In the end, you have to deal with the damage. "Nobody really has the power to make you eat more; only you can open your mouth and put food in it," says Ronna Kabatznick, Ph.D., psychologist and consultant to *Weight Watchers* magazine.

Although you and you alone decide what you eat and when, saying no to food pushers can be tricky. "You have to be vigilant, know what your emotional vulnerabilities are, and understand that eating is often connected to those times when you're feeling less strong or powerful," says Dr. Kabatznick. But, she adds, this is a terrific opportunity to practice standing up for yourself. Here's how to say no, graciously and firmly.

Practice assertiveness. To make things easier, use this four-step assertiveness process to get people to understand where you are coming from.

1. Describe the problem. How is the person hindering your fat-fighting efforts?
2. Express how you feel about the problem, without blaming the person.
3. Specify what you would like that person to do instead.
4. Explain the consequences of making that change.

You can say, for instance, "I've been trying to slim down. But every night before bed, you get a big bowl of ice cream and ask me if I want some. I have a hard time saying no to such temptation. It would really help my efforts if you wouldn't offer me the ice cream."

Persuade others to buy into your plan. Some people have a personal stake in your weight-loss plan. Your family may not want to eat low-fat, for instance, while you do. So think about all the people who may be affected by your weight-loss efforts. Then explain to them why this fat-fighting plan is so important to you, how you think it may affect them, and what you need them to do to help you out. Ask how you can make the process easier on them. And ask them to let you know when your efforts are really cramping their style, says Dr. Nash.

Compromise. Sometimes, you need to do more than express your feelings. You need to find a middle ground. If your family has absolutely no intention of eating "diet" food, for instance, strike a compromise. They could agree to buy their own fat-laden snacks and keep them somewhere in the house that you never enter. Or they could go out for fast food as long as they don't expect you to go along.

Outrun the Food Police

They watch the way you eat. They read the menu for you. They make faces and click their tongues when they see what you put in your grocery cart. They are the food police, imagined or self-appointed arbiters of your eating habits. They exist among the ranks of your friends, coworkers, and family—and some are even strangers. Your spouse or mother may be chief of the food police. And they make you feel guilty every time you eat.

So you eat on the sly, devouring hundreds or thousands of calories in a short period of time, says Connie Roberts, R.D., manager of nutrition consultation services and wellness programs at Brigham and Women's Hospital in Boston.

Recognizing the food police is easy. If you get a tense feeling in the pit of your stomach, a tightness every time you and someone else are around food together, trust it. That person is a food cop. And he or she is someone you want to either avoid or confront, says Dr. Olson. Here are some strategies.

Define what you need. Figure out exactly how you want others to treat you, and then tell them. Do you want them to

No More Nasty Thoughts

Depending on what you tell yourself, the ongoing dialogue about weight loss that takes place in your head can help or hinder your fat-fighting efforts, says Susan Olson, Ph.D., a clinical psychologist and weight-management consultant in Seattle and author of *Keeping It Off: Winning at Weight Loss*.

Here are some common sabotaging thoughts, along with alternatives to put you in the right mindset. According to Dr. Olson, these were originally identified by Michael J. and Kathryn Mahoney, authors of *Permanent Weight Control*.

When You Catch Yourself Thinking . . .	Tell Yourself Instead . . .
I'm not losing weight fast enough.	If I continue my healthy eating habits, I'll lose the weight eventually.
I've starved myself and haven't lost weight.	Those pounds took a long time to get there. I'll settle for any progress.

champion your successes and ignore your failures? Or do you wish they would never bring up the topic of food, exercise, or weight loss in your presence? For many people, the latter holds true. Explain that seemingly complimentary comments can pack a sting. You could start by describing that benign comments such as "Wow, I can see you've lost some weight" make you feel pressured to lose more, says Dr. Nash.

When You Catch Yourself Thinking . . .	Tell Yourself Instead . . .
I've been more consistent than my friend, who's losing weight faster. It's not fair.	Who says life has to be fair?
I don't have the willpower.	There's no such thing as willpower, just poor planning. Let's take 1 day at a time.
I'd be able to lose weight if it weren't for my (spouse/kids/job).	My schedule isn't any worse than other people's. I just need to be a bit more creative.
I get so nervous I have to eat.	Eating doesn't solve my psychological problems; it creates them.
I'm doomed to be fat just like my relatives.	If fat is an inheritance, I want it to be cut out of the will.
There goes my diet. That coffee cake just cost me 2 pounds.	What is this, the food Olympics? I don't need perfect habits, just improved ones. I'll cut back someplace else.

Rehearse those encounters you dread. Think about, act out, or even write out how confronting a food cop will turn out. Imagine what you are going to say. List the possible responses of the saboteur. Then decide how you will respond to each scenario, recommends Dr. Nash.

Tell them once, tell them twice, tell them again. "Sometimes, it takes more than one time of saying, 'Here's what

I need from you. Please don't watch over me. Please don't watch everything I eat. And please don't give me those looks,'" says Dr. Nash.

Keep a safe distance. "Sometimes, no matter how good you are at communicating your needs, particularly with mothers, they don't seem to get the message," says Dr. Nash. If necessary, limit the amount of time you spend together until you feel stronger about your efforts.

Take the Emphasis off Your Weight

The simple phrase "I'm trying to lose (blank) pounds" can be a huge pitfall. Even though you may do everything right—you eat low-fat, you exercise, and you practice portion control—the weight may not slide off as quickly as you'd like. You may occasionally hit plateaus. And so you say to yourself, "This isn't working"—and you quit.

When that happens, you tend to revert to eating high-fat foods and watching television, so you gain even more weight.

Instead of obsessing about every pound you lose or don't lose, you would do better to focus on the beneficial changes you are making that may eventually help you lose. In other words, focus on the process rather than the outcome. "Focusing on a weight number is a way to sabotage yourself. It really is better to focus on changing your habits," says Dr. Nash. Slowly cut back on the amount of fat in your diet, and slowly increase how much time you spend exercising. Then "let your weight fall where it may," says Dr. Nash.

If you have an intimate relationship with the bathroom scale—and find breaking off that relationship can be tougher than getting out of a dysfunctional love affair—try these strategies.

Go in small increments. If you still catch yourself taking a peek at your weight and continuing to set a weight-loss goal, try to break up your goal into small, manageable increments of 10 pounds or less. If you feel that you have 100 pounds to lose, for instance, focus on the first 10. Then, once you lose 10, focus on the next 10, says Dr. Nash. That way, you won't feel overwhelmed.

Talk to the scale. Your scale is your assistant, not your boss, your mother, or your guru. If the number you sneak a peek at today happens to be higher than the number you noticed the last time regardless of the fact that you've been eating sensibly and exercising in the interim, it may be because you drank more water than usual, because you consumed more water-retaining salt or monosodium glutamate, or because your menstrual period is here (or fast approaching). And while it's not fair, sometimes your weight goes up for no discernible reason at all.

The real questions to ask yourself as you hop on and off the scale are "How am I eating? How often am I exercising? How do I look? How do I feel?" The more you come up with answers you like, the more you'll realize that the number on the scale is just a number.

Tally your score. One way to focus on the process rather than the weight-loss goal is to track your food and activity habits. Tallying makes you aware of your habits and keeps your goals and your successes right there in front of you. Use a plain sheet of paper to track every activity you do (including things like taking the stairs instead of the elevator) and all the food that you eat (including the amounts). If you face a special challenge, put that on the paper too.

If one of your goals is to eat regular meals rather than pick at food all day, for instance, write down the time of each meal and snack (or try writing it beforehand). Once you are at your goal weight, you can try to keep track of food and activities mentally for a while. Just return to paper record keeping if you notice that your healthy habits are beginning to go astray.

Motivation Made Easy

The first few weeks on any weight-loss plan are the easiest, "but the honeymoon ends a few weeks into the attempt," says Susan J. Bartlett, Ph.D., associate director of clinical psychology at the Johns Hopkins Weight Management Center in Baltimore. So you make excuses. Or you cheat. Or you find yourself complaining.

And you fall off the weight-loss wagon.

The thing is, you can make that motivation-packed honeymoon last for the rest of your life. How? With careful planning.

Set Inspiring Goals

Quite possibly, motivation wanes because you have tied your goal to a number on the scale and get discouraged when you don't like what the scale tells you. First of all, scales can lie: Fluid shifts can hold the scale steady even though you have actually slimmed down. Second, like setting out for a distant destination without a map, setting a goal in itself offers no clues about how to get where you're going.

For more motivation, set a series of short-term goals that break your weight-loss task into achievable sections, giving you a strategy that leads to your long-term objective. Here's a breakdown of the characteristics that experts say your goals should have for best results.

They are achievable. Saying "I'll never eat sugar again" usually lands you in the pantry a week later with a handful of cookies and a big load of guilt, says Susan K. Rhodes, Ph.D., research associate in the department of psychiatry and behavioral sciences and director of research for the weight-management center at the Medical University of South Carolina College of Medicine in Charleston. A more realistic goal: For the next few weeks, put a reasonable number of cookies into your food plan.

They are specific. Effective goals define not only what you plan to do but how, where, and when you'll do it, such as "At least four times this week, I'm going to try to write down my meals before I eat them."

They are focused on behavior. Beware of the I'm-going-to-lose-a-pound-this-week trap. You can't guarantee yourself a weight change. What you can say is "I'm going to walk every day this week" or "I'm going to nibble on carrots rather than chocolate this week."

They are just a little beyond reach. A weight-loss goal that's too difficult will make you want to give up. A goal that's too easy may not get you anywhere. At first, set modest goals that you can achieve quickly, such as switching from whole milk to 2% or 1% milk. Then begin to set more ambitious goals, such as switching to fat-free milk.

Here's some other advice on how to set inspiring goals.

Reward yourself. You can choose anything for a reward as long as it is enjoyable, immediate, and available only when the goal is met. Some people do better if they reward themselves each time they accomplish a difficult task. They'll put a dollar in a jar after each exercise session, for instance, or allow themselves to soak in a hot tub for 30 minutes.

Think of at least 20 small, nonfood rewards for yourself. They should be simple, short-term things you would like to have or do that don't take a lot of time or money. Then write each one on a separate slip of paper and put the papers in an empty cookie jar. Each day, as you accomplish a mini-goal, draw from the reward jar.

Time your rewards. Instead of always rewarding yourself after the fact, find ways to reward yourself during an ac-

Quotes to Inspire You

When fighting fat gets tough, remember that even famous people struggle with weight. Here's what some well-known celebrities say about their personal weight-loss journeys.

Weight loss takes time, effort, desire, and arming yourself with tactics and education. It's about learning to use those elements that we know work, like fat reduction and portion control, and applying those to everyday cooking. It's about identifying your vulnerable points, your habits, what it is you're doing wrong, and then breaking those habits and replacing them with things you can do right—things that you enjoy!

—Joan Lunden in her book
Joan Lunden's Healthy Cooking

I am easier with myself these days, more forgiving, more content. I have learned, for example, that there is Life After Cellulite. When I'm in the company of a model, I don't wish to have her figure. I've got my own, and it's perfectly nice—it's me, after all.

—Sarah Ferguson, Duchess of York,
in her book *My Story*

tivity. If you like to watch *The Oprah Winfrey Show*, for instance, but you can't usually find the time, only allow yourself to partake while pedaling a stationary bike. Or reward yourself by watching a movie while you're on the treadmill or stationary bike.

Write it down. Seeing your goals on paper, where you can update them, will make them seem more real and boost your motivation to achieve them, says Virginia Bass, a time-management consultant and owner of By Design, a personal and professional development company in Exton, Pennsylvania, who teaches executives to do this

This new way of eating very low fat, low sugar, low salt (I like to call it clean eating) has made such a difference in my life. I feel better. But do not be misled: Changing the way you think about food is only the first step toward achieving and maintaining a desirable weight. It was only through a comprehensive plan of healthy eating, daily exercise, and changing my self-defeating behavior that I was able to release weight as an issue from my life.

—Oprah Winfrey in the book
In the Kitchen with Rosie

Food is one of the greatest pleasures in life. It is not your enemy! Yet most people approach the meal table with tension. I look forward to each and every meal. I know I'm going to eat wonderful food and enjoy the company of my friends and loved ones.

—Suzanne Somers in her book
Suzanne Somers' Eat Great, Lose Weight

for all kinds of goals. So put your mini-goals on paper, then give yourself a star once you accomplish them. Or make a formal contract with a buddy. Include your goal and the reward for reaching it.

See it happen. Close your eyes and visualize yourself accomplishing your week's goals. If your mini-goal is to get up 15 minutes earlier to walk the dog, for instance, in your mind see the alarm clock set at 6:15 A.M. instead of 6:30. See Spot at your bedside with his tail wagging. Your sweats and walking shoes are next to the bed, where you placed them the night before. Picture yourself getting into them and getting out there. Then you're set to really do it.

Maintaining Momentum

You can capitalize on the motivation you feel at the beginning of a weight-loss adventure by making some careful plans for later in your fat-fighting journey. Details to remember:

Do a cost–benefit analysis. Divide a sheet of paper into two vertical columns. In the left-hand column, list all the benefits of sticking to your weight-loss plan. Some examples are "I've already dropped 6 pounds," "I have more energy," "I deal with stress better." Under those items, jot down the costs of not sticking to the program, like "I'll be out of shape" or "My belly will come back."

In the right-hand column, write the costs of following your program, such as "I have to cut back on favorite foods that are loaded with fat" or "I have to make time for exercise." Then include the benefits of abandoning the program, such as "I'll have more time to myself because I won't be walking every day" or "I'll be able to eat and drink whatever I want."

"The things in the left column are the thoughts that will motivate you. When your thoughts start drifting to the right column, to the costs of making the changes and the benefits of not bothering, that undermines your motivation," says Joyce D. Nash, Ph.D., clinical psychologist in San Francisco and Palo Alto, California, and author of *The New Maximize Your Body Potential*. Post the list where you can see it every day, as both a visual and mental reminder. Being honest and open about your negative thoughts can help you figure out why you're starting to feel burned out, says Dr. Nash.

Check your records. At the beginning of your fat-fighting journey, write down your weight, body measurements, cholesterol levels, blood pressure, and any other vital statistics. Also write down the amount of time you spend exercising. Then later, if your motivation wanes, check out your progress. Avoid thinking about how far you have to go to reach your long-term weight-loss goals. Instead, pat yourself on the back for the progress that you have made.

Start for the right reasons. Perhaps you decide to lose weight because someone—spouse, mother, doctor—wants you to. Well, ignore them. "Trying to lose weight because others want you to creates a commitment that may cause feelings of resentment," says Dr. Bartlett, and resentment can weaken your resolve. Telling yourself that you "have to" or "should" lose weight, exercise, or stay away from particular foods brings up a rebellious twin that says, "I don't want to have to."

Write down all of the reasons that you decided to eat lower-fat foods and to exercise. Each sentence must start with the words "Because I choose to . . . ." When things occasionally get tough, refer to the list.

List your high-risk situations and your defense strategy. Maybe you tend to overeat at restaurants or you have an aversion to working out in cold weather or you have trouble stopping at just two nonfat oatmeal-raisin cookies.

Good Distractions

You're bored: You eat. You're depressed: You eat. You're stressed: You eat. You're mad: You eat.

Often, though, you can derail such behavior by doing something else to take your mind off your craving. Here are 20 things you can do to keep your mind off the high-fat food you crave.

1. Drink two glasses of water.
2. Brush your teeth and gargle.
3. Take a walk.
4. Take a nap.
5. Take a bath.
6. Call or write to the person who upset you.
7. Go to a movie.
8. Buy yourself a nonfood gift.
9. Have sex.
10. Snack on safe food such as an apple, rice cake, or carrot.
11. Call a friend.
12. Meditate.
13. Eat some fruit.
14. Leave the building for 10 minutes.
15. Play on the computer.
16. Catch up on office news with a coworker.
17. Walk to the watercooler, get a drink, and walk back.
18. Go to the rest room and splash cool water on your face.
19. Review your appointments for the upcoming week.
20. Walk up a few flights of stairs.

Write each of your most tempting situations on the fronts of index cards. Then think of as many counterstrikes as you can and note them on the backs of the cards. Some suggestions are drink a glass of water and have a carrot or celery stalk to take the edge off your hunger before you leave for the restaurant; try mall walking or gym workouts in the winter; buy individually wrapped snacks, such as nonfat granola and fruit bars, to keep you from going on a binge. With your defense at the ready, you'll be equipped to handle anything and stay motivated right to the weight-loss finish line.

Keep Going through the Tough Times

Once you are well into your fat-fighting plan, you may still experience some motivational peaks and valleys. Often, you can link dips to boredom. Here are ways to liven up your routine.

Go on a food safari. Instead of making yourself as miserable as possible by forcing yourself to eat the blandest low-fat foods you can find, think of eating low-fat as a food adventure. Try different recipes. Try different low-fat foods. One low-fat brand of cheese might be better than another. One vegetarian chili recipe may taste meatier than another. The key is to try.

Spice up your diet. Give your tastebuds a treat: Try a new, exotic fruit or vegetable, a different type of fish, or a new low-fat or nonfat product each week. Start an herb garden and add fresh sprigs of basil, oregano, cilantro, or parsley to your recipes. Every time you go to the grocery store, hunt down one new low-fat food that you've never tried before. It could be a frozen entrée or an exotic fruit.

Change your workout routine. Take your act on the road. Instead of stationary cycling, traverse wooded trails on a mountain bike. Walk in a new area or with a new partner. Try a workout in the morning instead of waiting until the afternoon. Take up a new sport or switch from weight-lifting machines to a free-weight workout.

Or experiment with interval training: After a 10- or 15-minute warmup, step up your pace for about 2 minutes. Slow down to catch your breath, recovering for about 1 minute, then speed up again for another 2. Vary your workouts as much as you like in order to keep them fresh and exciting.

Get a partner. Two exercisers are better than one. On those days when you feel like copping out, your partner can talk you into working out.

Break up your exercise session. Some people find exercise less boring if they break it up into numerous short sessions instead of one long, arduous workout. Try walking for 10 minutes before work, 15 minutes at lunch, and 10 minutes after dinner, for instance. It doesn't seem like a 35-minute workout, does it?

Distract yourself. Studies show that fast, upbeat music can help motivate you to exercise and keep you going longer. Other effective tactics include watching television or reading while working out on stationary equipment.

Holding Firm

Once you've lost all the weight you've planned to lose, you take on a new motivational challenge.

"During maintenance, there isn't that psychological reward of getting on the scale and seeing a smaller number," points out Judy E. Marshel, R.D., director of Health Resources in Great Neck, New York, and former senior nutritionist for Weight Watchers International. "Your goal is to see the same number all the time, and for some people it's not nearly as satisfying."

You can keep your motivation going strong, however, just by switching mental tracks. You no longer have a weight-loss goal but rather a lifestyle goal. Weight maintenance is a lifetime endeavor.

In order to stay motivated and value your efforts, look for new ways to pat yourself on the back. Each morning as you get dressed, for instance, remind yourself how well your clothes fit. Or each time you get on the scale and the number has not budged, consider the event a cause for celebration. You may have completed the weight-loss race, but now you are embarking on a new, more challenging adventure.

A Sensible Program Takes Time and Patience

At the University of Alabama at Birmingham's EatRight weight-loss center, coordinator Beth Bussey, R.D., won't let women lose more than 10 percent of their weight within 3 months. If the women start to lose weight too quickly, Bussey tells them to eat more.

At that pace, fat fighting doesn't even seem worth the time spent exercising, reading labels, or shopping for nostick cookware. In reality, however, weight that comes off as slow as molasses is weight that will stay off. So if you're in a fat-fighting rush, heed these reasons for losing fat slowly.

• While you could initially lose weight faster by severely restricting your food intake, you'll have a harder time reaching your goal weight. Eating too few calories slows your metabolism, the rate at which your body burns calories, causing a weight-loss plateau. So regardless of how few calories you eat, your weight essentially remains stagnant well before you hit your goal.

• Rapid weight loss usually brings on plumper returns. Once you start eating more food after ending a low-calorie diet, you gain weight faster than before you began dieting because your metabolism isn't burning calories as well. Then every time you crash diet to get rid of this new fat, your metabolism slows down even more quickly, which makes weight loss even harder.

• If you restrict calories long enough, your basal metabolic rate can drop to as low as 500 calories a day. When your body burns so few calories, you may feel cold, even in the summer. You may also feel tired and notice other side effects, such as dry skin, constipation, and depression. A super-low diet can also pose significant health risks such as heartbeat irregularities and mineral imbalances, which can be life threatening.

• Another potential by-product of rapid weight loss is also a painful one: gallstones. Usually, the gallbladder contracts to empty itself of bile and cholesterol. When food intake is low, however, the gallbladder loses its ability to contract, so cholesterol is more likely to build up and thicken into painful gallstones.

To get over the urge to crash diet and shed those pounds fast, try to focus instead on the tons of lifestyle changes that you are making. Reward yourself for making the switch from whole milk to fat-free, for instance. Pat yourself on the back for eating breakfast. Give yourself a high five for walking in the morning. The more you focus on the small external changes you make to lose weight, the less you'll obsess about how much weight you are losing and how fast.

Fitting in Weight Loss

You may think that cooking healthy food and exercising take too much time. That's not true.

For one thing, exercise actually creates time. After the first week or so of a regular exercise program, many people report that their levels of energy and stamina surge to the point where they feel as if they've actually gained extra productive hours in each day. Exercise also helps you gain time in the most literal sense: By reducing your risk of heart disease, osteoporosis, and other life-threatening diseases, you can add days and even years to your life.

Still, you'll be more likely to stick with your fat-fighting habits if you learn to fit them into your schedule. Here's how.

Plan your attack. Smart cooking begins with a plan, says Judy Gilliard, author of *The Guiltless Gourmet* and other cookbooks, who started to cook healthier meals when she was diagnosed with diabetes.

"We don't always have time to prepare food, so we make unhealthy choices, like grabbing a doughnut for breakfast. The key is to take a little time each week to pre-plan what we'll cook," says Suzanne Havala, R.D., a nutritionist in Charlotte, North Carolina, and author of *Simple, Lowfat and Vegetarian*.

Devote part of a weekend or other convenient time to planning your meals and making a shopping list, Gilliard suggests. Select healthier recipes that you'd like to try.

Reorganize your pantry. If your foods aren't where you can easily find them, you'll waste time hunting when you could be cooking, says Gilliard. "Group your canned tomato products—tomato sauce, tomato puree, stewed tomatoes, and the like—in one logical, convenient place, for instance. Do the same with canned beans, grains, oils, condiments, and so forth."

Out with the old. Go through your refrigerator, cabinets, and pantry and clean them out, says Gilliard. "Get rid of high-fat items and old items."

Presoak rice. To reduce the cooking time of regular brown rice, soak it overnight, says Marian Burros, who writes the "Eating Well" column for the *New York Times* and is the author of several books, including *Eating Well Is the Best Revenge*. Then, when you want to prepare it the next day, it will cook as quickly as white rice.

Leave the chopping to someone else. Take advantage of timesaving precut fresh produce at the supermarket, such as broccoli florets, carrot coins, watermelon cubes, and pineapple spears, as well as bags of frozen vegetables.

Save the work for a rainy day. On a blustery, rainy, or generally dreary day, prepare several low-fat, freeze-ahead meals and save yourself cooking time later in the week.

Walk and talk. Time that you usually spend chatting on the telephone, over lunch, or across a desk may provide an opportunity for fitness. Whether it's an intimate tête-à-tête with a good friend or a brainstorming session for an annual fund-raiser, consider carrying on the conversation while you walk for fitness. And if that means taking along a portable phone, so be it.

Improve your mind. Get fit while you get the news: Ride a stationary bike while reading the paper or watching CNN.

Shop for fitness. If you leave the car at home, you can turn hauling home a few groceries into an effective workout. Make sure your groceries are fairly evenly divided between two handled bags when you leave the store. Grab one in each hand and, as you walk, raise and lower the bags by bending your elbows one at a time or, better yet, at the same time. When your arms get tired, simply carry the bags normally for a block or two. Repeat until you get home.

Exercise on the go. Is traveling a big part of your job? Make those pockets of time work for you and your fitness regimen. Plan on getting to your destination 30 to 60 minutes early so you can use the hotel gym or jogging path. Stuck at the airport between planes? Do a couple of brisk laps around the terminal.

Play to your preferences. Combine fun with a physical challenge. Do you love to shop? Forget the TV shopping channels. Instead, fitness walk through your favorite shopping district before the stores open and preview the window displays. Got the travel bug? Sign up for a fitness-oriented vacation. Are you crafty by nature? Then take a nature walk and collect pinecones, twigs, and other found objects for your next project. Try all kinds of activities— bird-watching, gardening, table tennis, horseback riding, or social dancing. The best workouts aren't necessarily the ones that deliver the greatest calorie burn; rather, they're the activities that you're more likely to do because you honestly enjoy them.

Make Time, without Guilt

Here are some ways you can make time for exercise and other fat-fighting habits without feeling the tiniest pang of guilt, according to Virginia Bass, a time-management consultant and owner of By Design, a personal and professional development company in Exton, Pennsylvania.

Give the TV a rest. If you are watching for a few hours a day, your television time could be the easiest spot to cut back. You don't have to give up television for good. Just stick with your favorite shows and click off the tube when you realize that you are merely vegetating.

Get out of bed. You can create more time by getting up a few minutes earlier in the morning. Set your alarm a ½ hour to an hour earlier, then get up and go for a walk.

Let your timesaving devices do the job. Do you wash your dishes before sticking them in the dishwasher? Look for ways to use such appliances so that you can shave a minute here and a minute there off your preparation and

Buy a pedometer. To keep track of the distance you're covering in your daily walks, buy a pedometer (available for less than $20 at many sporting goods stores), suggests Judith S. Stern, R.D., Sc.D., professor of nutrition and internal medicine at the University of California at Davis. Aim for at least 4 miles a day, she says. If you go on vacation, pack your pedometer along with your walking shoes. Holidays often mean added indulgence, so try to increase your walking to offset the extra food, says Dr. Stern. If you're at the beach or in the country, you'll have lots of opportunities for outdoor walking. But even if it's a city vacation, you can cover plenty of ground by visiting museums and other sites of interest.

cleanup time in the kitchen. "It's very important to look for where minutes can be shaved," Bass says.

Take a shorter shower. Sure it feels good to stand under that stream of hot water while you daydream about who-knows-what for 5 to 10 minutes. But do you have to? If you normally take a 15-minute shower, try reducing it to 10 minutes. Over the course of 1 week, that small change will give you a ½ hour to spend exercising or planning healthy meals.

Say no to time sappers. You might refuse altogether: "No, I can't do that for you." You might reschedule: "No, I can't do that right now because I'm on my way to the gym. How about next week?" And you might compromise: "No, I can't host the holiday dinner. But I could bake a couple of pies."

Ask for help. Free up some time for yourself by sharing the chores with others. Even time spent on simple tasks like making the beds in the morning, clearing the table after dinner, or unloading the dishwasher can add up.

Be creative. "Did you know that during a typical ½-hour TV show, there are between 8 and 10 minutes of commercials? Use that time," says Dr. Stern. "When a commercial comes on, get up off the couch and walk around the house. Every time you do that, you get in an extra few minutes of exercise. You notice that I'm not saying to stop watching TV, just to make the most of it. The idea is to build good habits. The hope is that when exercise opportunities, such as taking stairs, present themselves, you'll automatically take advantage of them."

Have your stuff handy. Nothing can derail your intentions faster than sneakers that are still soggy from the weekend hike or personal-stereo batteries that are so run-down they make Frank Sinatra sound like Lurch from the Addams family. Flatten those paper tiger obstacles by keeping your gear ready to roll and, above all, handy. If you have to trip over your walking shoes on your way out the door, you're one step closer to leaving with them on.

Hitch exercise to an essential. Attaching exercise to something you absolutely have to do every day boosts your chances of doing it. Some exercisers leave the house without showering so they have to go to the gym on their way to work. Think about the things you can't live without and learn to use them to your fitness advantage.

Spare Time You Didn't Know You Had

Every day, we waste time—lots of it. If you take advantage of all of that time, cooking healthy foods and exercising won't seem so time-consuming. Here's how to round up some extra time.

Keep a time log. For about a week, write down how you've spent your time. This gives you a way to tell at a glance what occupies your day. Then look for tasks that are expendable or that you can at least cut back.

Do first things first. People often mistake activity for productivity. But simply by spending too much time on frivolous tasks, you can be very busy and still not get anything important done. Every Sunday, make a list for the week of things that need to be done or that you'd simply like to do. Choose the five most important items on the list and schedule time for them. Then arrange the less important tasks around those five. Finally, add the things you'd like to do if any time remains. Even if you don't follow through on everything, the five most important items will likely be taken care of. (And if being healthy and feeling good are important to you, don't forget to include exercise among your top priorities.)

Never do one thing when you can do two. Keep a magnetic note board on your refrigerator and maintain an ongoing list of errands. Before leaving the house, check your list to see if there isn't some way to combine two or more of them.

Buy several generic greeting cards. If someone has a baby, you need to go out and buy a baby card. Someone has a birthday—another visit to the card shop. Forget it. Make one trip and buy 10 attractive cards that have no preprinted message inside. Keep the cards with some stamped envelopes and simply reach for one when you need it, penning inscriptions appropriate to the occasion.

Make haircuts a breeze. Many chains, such as Supercuts or Holiday Hair, offer walk-in service that requires no appointment. But if you don't want to waste time reading outdated magazines while waiting for a chair, the best time to go is Monday through Wednesday between 1:00 and 4:00 in the afternoon. Avoid weekends before the three busiest haircutting times of the year: Mother's Day, Easter, and before the kids go back to school in the fall.

Box it. Somewhere between no filing system at all and one that's so meticulous that it takes an hour a day to maintain, there's a simpler way to never lose another piece of paper: the three-box system. Keep one box to toss bills into, another for recipes and coupons, and a third for miscellaneous stuff that you don't need right now but probably will soon. Once a month, go through the boxes. Pay the bills, use the coupons, and throw out what you don't need.

Hire help. While a live-in maid, a full-time gardener, and a cook might be a bit pricier than most of us can afford, there's no reason you can't hire some occasional help when it's less expensive than doing it yourself. The rule of thumb is this: Figure out what your time is worth by calculating your hourly rate at the office. If you make $20 an hour and little Timmy down the street will rake your leaves for $5, that's a bargain.

Make your next appointment during your current one. You know you'll need another haircut in 8 weeks, so why not make the appointment while you're at the salon for a trim? The same thing applies to dental appointments, physicals, and even automotive tune-ups.

Put things back where you found them. Sure, it's one of the oldest tricks in the book—so old that nobody seems to pay it any mind. To see just how much simpler life could be when it's orderly, compare the amount of time it takes to consistently hang your car keys on a nail beside the front door with the amount of time, anger, and cussing it takes to try to find them under a couch cushion or by the phone.

Get a cordless phone. Around the house, having a cordless phone means uninterrupted conversations while walking on the treadmill, chopping vegetables, or even cleaning the fridge.

Let your grass grow. You can waste a lot of time and sweat cutting your grass more than necessary. The optimal grass length is 2½ to 3 inches in the summer. That allows the grass to grow more slowly. Whenever you cut grass shorter, it shoots up at the fastest rate possible. Also, at the recommended length, your lawn will become dense enough to crowd out weeds, reducing the need for you to crawl on your hands and knees to pull dandelions.

Shop at the right time. In general, you'll find the smallest number of shopping lines on Tuesday and Wednesday. But even those days have their rush periods. Peak daily times include the lunch hour and the hours between 4:30 and 7:30 P.M., when the office crowd does its shopping.

Use automatic deposit. There's no need for you to drag a paycheck over to the bank, write slips, and stand in line. Your company's payroll department will probably be happy to set up a direct deposit system for you.

Index

Underscored page references indicate boxed text.